Pediatric Headaches: Diagnostic and Therapeutic Issues

Pediatric Headaches: Diagnostic and Therapeutic Issues

Guest Editor

Alberto Maria Cappellari

MDPI

Basel • Beijing • Wuhan • Barcelona • Belgrade • Novi Sad • Cluj • Manchester

Guest Editor
Alberto Maria Cappellari
Department of Neuroscience
and Mental Health
Fondazione IRCCS Ca' Granda
Ospedale Maggiore
Policlinico
Milan
Italy

Editorial Office
MDPI AG
Grosspeteranlage 5
4052 Basel, Switzerland

This is a reprint of the Special Issue, published open access by the journal *Children* (ISSN 2227-9067), freely accessible at: https://www.mdpi.com/journal/children/special_issues/2Q5L9IMAF3.

For citation purposes, cite each article independently as indicated on the article page online and as indicated below:

Lastname, A.A.; Lastname, B.B. Article Title. *Journal Name* **Year**, *Volume Number*, Page Range.

ISBN 978-3-7258-6688-5 (Hbk)
ISBN 978-3-7258-6689-2 (PDF)
https://doi.org/10.3390/books978-3-7258-6689-2

Contents

About the Editor vii

Preface ix

Salvatore Di Marco, Laura Pilati, Angelo Torrente, Simona Maccora, Andrea Santangelo, Giuseppe Cosentino, et al.
Pediatric Migraine and Visual Cortical Excitability: A Prospective Observational Study with Sound-Induced Flash Illusions
Reprinted from: *Children* **2024**, *11*, 394, https://doi.org/10.3390/children11040394 1

Allison M. Smith, Megan N. Silvia, Hannah Rogan and Alyssa A. Lebel
The Photo- and Phonosensitivity Avoidance Behavior Scales: Evaluating Clinical Utility in Pediatric Primary Chronic Headache
Reprinted from: *Children* **2024**, *11*, 1338, https://doi.org/10.3390/children11111338 13

Seung Beom Han, Eu Gene Park and Ji Yoon Han
Clinical and Multivariate Predictors of Headaches Attributed to Rhinosinusitis in Pediatric Patients: A Comparative Study with Migraine and Tension-Type Headache
Reprinted from: *Children* **2025**, *12*, 1557, https://doi.org/10.3390/children12111557 27

Samantha Glover, Linda Sangalli and Caroline M. Sawicki
Training, Awareness, and Clinical Perspectives of Pediatric Dentists on Headache and Migraine Management: A National Survey Study
Reprinted from: *Children* **2025**, *12*, 968, https://doi.org/10.3390/children12080968 44

Alberto M. Cappellari, Gaia Bruschi, Gisella B. Beretta, Maria T. Molisso and Giuseppe Bertolozzi
How Can Specialist Advice Influence the Neuroimaging Practice for Childhood Headache in Emergency Department?
Reprinted from: *Children* **2023**, *10*, 1837, https://doi.org/10.3390/children10121837 58

Jacob Genizi, Lotan Berger, Muhammad Mahajnah, Yulia Shlonsky, Orit Golan-Shany, Azriel Romem, et al.
High CCL2 Levels Detected in CSF of Patients with Pediatric Pseudotumor Cerebri Syndrome
Reprinted from: *Children* **2023**, *10*, 1122, https://doi.org/10.3390/children10071122 68

Corinna Börner-Schröder, Magdalena Lang, Giada Urban, Erik Zaidenstadt, Jacob Staisch, Ari Hauser, et al.
Neuromodulation in Pediatric Migraine Using Repetitive Neuromuscular Magnetic Stimulation: A Feasibility Study
Reprinted from: *Children* **2023**, *10*, 1764, https://doi.org/10.3390/children10111764 74

Amit Blumovich, Trevor Gerson, Mark Connelly, Tammie Wingert and Gina Jones
The Real-World Evaluation of Remote Electrical Neuromodulation in Pediatric Migraines: A Preliminary Study
Reprinted from: *Children* **2025**, *12*, 1500, https://doi.org/10.3390/children12111500 91

Dimitrios Panagopoulos, Maro Gavra, Efstathios Boviatsis, Stefanos Korfias and Marios Themistocleous
Chronic Pediatric Headache as a Manifestation of Shunt Over-Drainage and Slit Ventricle Syndrome in Patients Harboring a Cerebrospinal Fluid Diversion System: A Narrative Literature Review
Reprinted from: *Children* **2024**, *11*, 596, https://doi.org/10.3390/children11050596 98

About the Editor

Alberto Maria Cappellari

Alberto Maria Cappellari is a doctor of neurology at the Department of Neuroscience and Mental Health of Fondazione IRCCS Ca' Granda Ospedale Maggiore Policlinico, Milan, Italy. His clinical and research activity is focused on several fields of pediatric neurology, including epilepsy, headache, movement disorders, and neuromuscular diseases.

Preface

Headache is one of the most common symptoms in children and adolescents and can cause significant distress in patients and their families. Headaches can also be worrisome for clinicians, owing to the variety of underlying etiologies, both benign and serious.

In recent years, there have been several advances in the understanding of the pathophysiology, assessment, and management of migraine and other headaches.

In the Special Issue "Pediatric Headaches: Diagnostic and Therapeutic Issues", we aim to update the knowledge on headaches in children and adolescents by presenting a collection of articles from authors across the world that address both clinical and research issues. The first section begins with articles focusing on sensory phenomena associated with headache, such as sound-induced flash illusions in pediatric migraine and photo- and phonosensitivity in pediatric primary chronic headache. This is followed by articles discussing the involvement of different specialists in the management of pediatric headaches, including the analysis of predictors of headaches attributed to rhinosinusitis and awareness of the link between oral conditions and headaches. Then, specific investigation issues are considered, such as the influence of specialist advice on the neuroimaging practice for childhood headache in the emergency department and the preliminary evidence of a potential pathogenetic marker in the cerebrospinal fluid of children with pseudotumor cerebri. Finally, later articles in this Issue discuss some non-pharmacological modalities for treatment of pediatric migraine, including neuromodulation using repetitive neuromuscular magnetic stimulation and remote electrical neuromodulation, and the management of headache related to shunt over-drainage and slit ventricle syndrome, which is secondary to the surgical treatment of pediatric hydrocephalus.

The Special Issue "Pediatric Headaches: Diagnostic and Therapeutic Issues" is addressed to many clinicians involved in the management of pediatric headaches in clinical practice (pediatricians, neurologists, child neuropsychiatrists, neurosurgeons, otolaryngologists, and other healthcare specialists), as well as trainees (students, residents, and fellows). It is our hope that this issue further stimulates ongoing research in the field of pediatric headaches.

We would like to thank the authors who participated in this Special Issue for their valuable contributions.

Alberto Maria Cappellari
Guest Editor

children

MDPI

Article

Pediatric Migraine and Visual Cortical Excitability: A Prospective Observational Study with Sound-Induced Flash Illusions

Salvatore Di Marco [1,2], Laura Pilati [1,2], Angelo Torrente [1], Simona Maccora [1,3], Andrea Santangelo [4], Giuseppe Cosentino [5,6], Edvige Correnti [7], Vincenzo Raieli [7,*], Brigida Fierro [1] and Filippo Brighina [1]

1 Department of Biomedicine, Neuroscience and advanced Diagnostics (BiND), University of Palermo, 90127 Palermo, Italy; dimarcosal@gmail.com (S.D.M.); laura.pilati.91@gmail.com (L.P.); angelo.torrente@unipa.it (A.T.); simona.maccora@unipa.it (S.M.); brigida.fierro@unipa.it (B.F.); filippo.brighina@unipa.it (F.B.)
2 Neurology and Stroke Unit, P.O. "S. Antonio Abate", 91016 Trapani, Italy
3 Neurology Unit, ARNAS Civico di Cristina and Benfratelli Hospitals, 90127 Palermo, Italy
4 Pediatrics Department, AOUP Santa Chiara Hospital, 56126 Pisa, Italy; a.santangelo9@studenti.unipi.it
5 Translational Neurophysiology Research Unit, IRCCS Mondino Foundation, 27100 Pavia, Italy; giuseppe.cosentino@unipv.it
6 Department of Brain and Behavioral Sciences, University of Pavia, 27100 Pavia, Italy
7 Child Neurology and Psychiatry Unit—ISMEP, "G. Di Cristina" Children's Hospital—ARNAS Civico, 90127 Palermo, Italy; edvige.correnti@arnascivico.it
* Correspondence: vincenzo.raieli@arnascivico.it

Abstract: The pathophysiological mechanisms underlying migraine are more difficult to investigate in children than in the adult population. Abnormal cortical excitability turns out to be one of the most peculiar aspects of migraine, accounting for the manifestations of migraine attacks. Recently, visual cortical excitability has been explored effectively in adult migraineurs with a technique based on cross-modal audio-visual illusions (with sound-induced flash illusions (SIFIs) being reduced in migraineurs compared to non-migraineur subjects). On such a basis, in this study, we investigated visual cortical excitability in children with migraine using SIFIs using combinations of visual and sound stimuli presented randomly. We evaluated 26 children with migraine without aura and 16 healthy children. Migraineurs did not differ from the age-matched healthy subjects regarding fission or fusion illusions but perceived more flashes in trials of multiple flashes with or without beeps. The higher number of SIFIs in migraineur children compared to adults may be due to a greater propensity of visual stimulation to be driven by auditory stimuli (i.e., acoustic dominance). The increased ability to perceive flashes reveals a hyperfunctional visual cortex, demonstrating that the use of SIFIs is a valid tool for assessing visual cortical responsiveness even in pediatric migraine.

Keywords: pediatric migraine; cortical excitability; sound-induced flash illusion; headache

1. Introduction

Migraine is one of the most common forms of primary headache occurring during childhood [1]. About 1 out of 10 children suffer from migraine, even in the population under 7 years of age [2,3]. Migraine is considered an episodic and familial disorder characterized by recurrent headache episodes, widely varying in frequency, duration, and intensity. Furthermore, in adults, it is often responsible for relevant disability and high social and economic costs, in terms of healthcare expenditure (i.e., direct costs), loss of working days, and reduced productivity (i.e., indirect costs) [4]. An Italian study that investigated pediatric headache populations over six months found direct costs per child with migraine of EUR 802.80; moreover, the total indirect cost due to headache in the whole pediatric population was EUR 1323.30, with an average indirect cost per patient of EUR 52.97 (even considering parental work productivity loss) [5]. In addition to the linked societal costs, migraine represents one of the most associated causes of absenteeism from school [6].

During a migraine attack, the pain is usually accompanied by other symptoms such as nausea, pallor, phonophobia, and photophobia; moreover, in around a quarter of migraine patients, pain episodes are preceded or accompanied by transient focal neurologic symptoms, known as aura. Despite migraine usually being thought of as a disorder characterized by phasic transient cephalic pain episodes, the current knowledge is that it follows a cyclic pattern, with different phases. This "migraine cycle" sees (i) a pre-ictal (or prodromal) phase that may last up to 48 h before the attack, during which the patient experiences non-specific symptoms such as yawning, mood changes, or food craving; (ii) ictal phase represented by the headache and its associated symptoms; (iii) a post-ictal (or post-dromal) phase that may last up to 48 h and include other non-specific symptoms such as tiredness and fluid retention; and (iiii) an interictal phase between each post-dromal phase and the next pre-ictal phase [7–9]. Even though the interictal phase may be a headache-free time, several patients still experience some symptoms including subjective memory impairment, psychological symptoms, or constant photo- or phonophobia.

In childhood, there are, in addition, some heterogeneous clinical signs related to migraines such as infant colic, abdominal migraine, cyclic vomiting, and benign paroxysmal vertigo, once considered possible precursors of the disease (i.e., migraine equivalent) [1,10]. Differently from the adult form, pediatric migraine is characterized by attacks of a shorter duration, less pronounced lateralization [11], and an aura that may be atypical [12], and it may be accompanied by cranial autonomic disturbances [13]. In addition, migraineur children may present a different response to preventive drugs from adults [2].

The human brain shows a maturation that extends over time, and the developmental trajectories are different in different brain structures, neural circuits, and white matter. These dynamic changes are particularly relevant during the developmental age. For instance, longitudinal MRI studies in healthy children have shown progressive increases in white matter, reversed trajectories of grey matter, and increased connectivity in adolescence, while in developmental pathologies, changes in these typical trajectories can be observed [14,15]. For these and various other reasons, the child cannot be considered a small adult, especially from a neurological point of view [16].

Despite the large body of literature focused on this area, migraine etiopathogenesis has not yet been fully understood, but consistent evidence emphasizes the role of abnormalities of cortical excitability [17,18]. There are forms of migraine (familial hemiplegic migraine—FHM) in which the pathogenetic mutation depends on genes of some particular channel proteins involved in normal neuronal functioning and the control of cortical excitability [19,20]. Knock-in mice for these mutated genes showed a greater susceptibility to developing cortical spreading depression (CSD), a phenomenon considered to be the basis of migraine aura [21].

An important contribution to the evaluation of cortical abnormalities in migraine comes from studies based on neurophysiological investigations such as evoked potentials and non-invasive brain stimulation (NIBS) techniques like transcranial magnetic stimulation (TMS) and transcranial direct current stimulation (tDCS). These techniques revealed abnormal cortical excitability in migraine, particularly in the visual cortex [21,22]. Such results, suggesting that migraineurs show increased cortical excitability, have been supported both by studies with repetitive TMS (rTMS) and with a paired-pulse paradigm [23]. Even the phosphene threshold (PT, i.e., the lowest TMS intensity to induce the perception of phosphenes in a subject) was found altered in migraineurs. In basal conditions, they showed a reduced PT (reflecting an increased cortical excitability). Nevertheless, after an inhibitory low-frequency rTMS protocol on the occipital cortex, migraineurs seemed to have a paradoxical facilitatory effect, in contrast to the inhibitory effect on controls [24].

The excitability linked to the activation level of the occipital cortex plays an important role in the mechanisms of visual perception and the neural processes underlying cross-modal perception (i.e., the increased signal resulting from the interaction between two different sensory modalities). This phenomenon can be investigated by evaluating specifically induced illusory phenomena. One of the most used models is represented by sound-induced flash illusions (SIFIs), elaborated by Shams et al. to evaluate the audio-visual interaction of visual stimuli presented concurrently with auditory ones [25]. With this technique, when a single flash is accompanied by two or more beeps, the subject perceives more flashes than real ones (fission illusions); differently, fusion illusions arise when multiple flashes are presented with a single beep and are perceived as less than their real number. Even if the precise mechanisms underlying SIFIs remain to be defined, a critical role seems to be played by visual cortical excitability [26]. In 2011, Bolognini et al. [26] showed that artificially increasing the excitability of the occipital cortex through anodic facilitatory tDCS reduces the illusory phenomena. Considering the role of alterations in visual cortical excitability in migraine, Brighina et al. [27] evaluated the development of auditory-visual illusions in a group of adult migraine patients with and without aura, both in the interictal and in the ictal phases, and comparing data with healthy subjects. The results showed that in the case of fission illusion, all the subpopulations of migraineurs showed fewer illusions than controls. In this study, the cross-modal illusions were therefore demonstrated to be a valuable tool for exploring the functional connectivity between the sensory areas, which probably plays an important role in migraine pathophysiology [27].

During childhood, despite multisensory abilities already being present, as demonstrated by Innes-Brown et al. [28], the audio-visual illusory phenomenon is significantly increased compared to adults. This suggests that the selective integration ability of bimodal stimuli requires a very long period to develop completely (until late adolescence) [28]. Nava et al. [29] showed that the number of fission illusions presents a reduction trend with increasing age. This result may be correlated to the progressive maturation of multisensory integration systems during development, which sees the transition from an auditory dominance to a progressive visual one at an evolutionary age, implicating more and more emphasis on visual stimulation [29].

In the present study, the primary aim is to use SIFIs to evaluate the perception of the illusory auditory-visual phenomena in migraineur children compared with healthy controls in the same age range, to understand the role of abnormal excitability as related to basic pathophysiological mechanisms or as a marker of disease progression. Indeed, we hypothesized that as compared to healthy children, those affected by migraine would show a reduced extent of illusions, which means a condition of cortical hyperexcitability, as is found in adult migraineurs [30].

2. Materials and Methods

2.1. Participants

We enrolled pediatric subjects with migraine without aura diagnosed following the International Classification of Headache Disorders, third edition beta version (ICHD-3 beta) [31] criteria, with appropriate age-related variations. As inclusion criteria, children should have shown unremarkable neurological examination, no other comorbidities, normal or corrected vision by using graduated lenses, and normal hearing and should not have been undergoing any chronic or continuous pharmacological treatment. We also enrolled healthy subjects with the same age and sex distribution. During the inclusion, we also paid attention to avoiding the presence or any family medical history of migraine (among healthy children) or other neurological and psychiatric disorders (among all the subjects), which would have represented exclusion criteria.

All patients were examined during the interictal phase of the migraine cycle (i.e., at least 48 h after the last attack), and we checked for the absence of any new attack in the 48 h after the test through a telephone call. We performed the study only in patients affected by migraine without aura. This is because our principal aim was to explore the changes in cortical excitability related to migraine itself independently using cortical abnormalities linked to the mechanisms underlying aura. Moreover, migraine with aura presents a minor prevalence compared to migraine without aura, and considering the difficulties of recruiting pediatric patients, this aspect could have further reduced the chances of obtaining adequate populations for comparison.

The study was approved by the Palermo 1 Ethics Committee (Palermo, Italy, protocol no. 5/2015 of 13 May 2015), and the children underwent the test after both the parents received adequate information and signed a specific informed consent. The inclusion period was from June 2015 to March 2017. Migraine patients were recruited from the ones referring to the pediatric headache center of Di Cristina Hospital, while healthy subjects were in a class of catechism in Palermo, Italy.

2.2. Stimulation and Task

The participants sat in a dark room in front of a black screen located about 70 cm distance from their eyes. We used E-prime software (version 2.0®, Psychology Software Tools, Pittsburgh, PA, USA) to present, in random order, visual stimuli as white flash disks and sound stimuli with the following characteristics: sound intensity of 95 dB, frequency of 3.5 kHz, duration of 7 msec, and administered 23 msec before the flash. We distinguished between single-flash trials and multiple-flash trials. In single-flash trials, the flash (F) was accompanied by 0 to 4 beeps (B) (i.e., 1F0B, 1F1B, 1F2B, 1F3B, 1F4B, where 1F2B, 1F3B, and 1F4B trials aimed to induce the fission illusions); in multiple-flash trials, 2 to 4 flashes were accompanied by 0 to 1 beep (i.e., 2F0B, 3F0B, 4F0B, 2F1B, 3F1B, 4F1B, where 2F1B, 3F1B, and 4F1B trials aimed to induce the fusion illusions). Thus, the total number of combinations was 11. The task of the subjects was to fix the center of the screen and judge the number of flashes seen during each trial (see Figure 1). Each condition was repeated 10 times for a total of 110 randomly placed trials. Before the experiment was executed, 10 random non-recorded trials were presented to train the participants. The duration of a single experiment was 10 min.

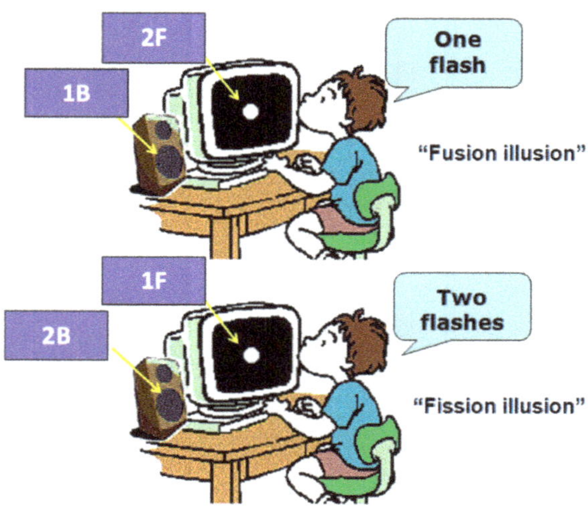

Figure 1. Simplification of the task required from the subjects.

2.3. Statistical Analysis

Supposing a normal distribution of data (later confirmed by a Shapiro–Wilk test), quantitative variables were presented as mean ± standard deviation (SD). Qualitative data were presented as % frequency. For the statistical analysis, the SIFI results for children with migraine were compared through analyses of variance (ANOVA) to evaluate the variability inside a group (ANOVA with repeated measures) and between groups (ANOVA between). To evaluate the hypothesis that children with migraine show a reduction of illusion, we compared SIFIs in healthy children to children with migraine.

3. Results

We studied 26 migraine patients (14 males, 12 females) with an age of 11.30 ± 2.43 years. These were compared with 16 healthy subjects (8 males, 8 females) with an age of 10.61 ± 2.92 years. Among the female subjects, 7/12 (58.33%) patients and 3/8 (37.50%) healthy children had already started to have their period. Among the overall patients, the mean monthly migraine days were 4.31 ± 2.33, and the diagnosis had been performed from 34.42 ± 23.37 months; they did not show symptoms during the interictal period. Table 1 summarizes the patients' clinical characteristics.

Table 1. Migraine population clinical characteristics.

Variable	Mean	SD
Migraine frequency (days/month)	4.31	2.33
Months since diagnosis	34.42	23.37
Headache intensity (NRS)	7.50	1.45
Attack duration (hours)	5.96	6.31

Abbreviations: NRS = numeric rating scale; SD = standard deviation.

3.1. Singe-Flash Trials

We performed an ANOVA with two factors: (i) conditions—single-flash trials with one flash and 0 to 4 beeps (five levels: 1F0B, 1F1B, 1F2B, 1F3B, 1F4B), and (ii) group (two levels: healthy subjects and migraineurs), which showed the following results (see Figure 2 and Table 2). In the interaction group for conditions: F (4, 160) = 0.42156, p = 0.79292; in the condition factor: F (4, 160) = 124.29, p = 0.00001; and in the group factor: F (1, 40) = 1.0179, p = 0.31907.

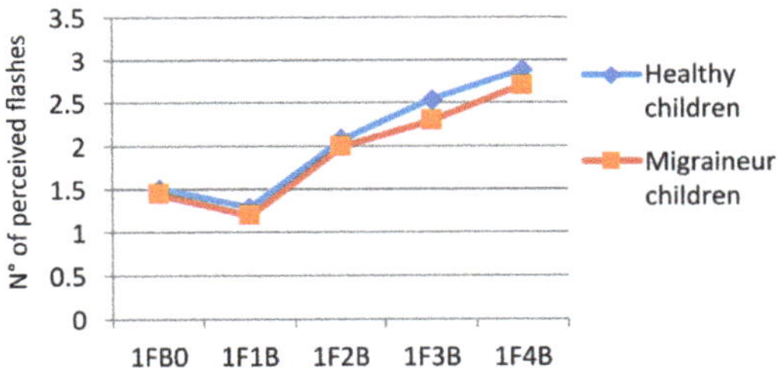

Figure 2. Fission illusions in children with migraine and healthy children during single-flash trials. On the x-axis, the flashes (F) and beeps (B) combination of the different trials are given: for example, 1FB0 means the presentation of one flash and no beep. On the y-axis, the mean number of perceived flashes is reported.

Table 2. Single-flash trial results.

Test	Group	Mean	SD
1FB0	HC	1.51	0.396
	MC	1.44	0.403
1F1B	HC	1.29	0.403
	MC	1.20	0.251
1F2B	HC	2.08	0.650
	MC	1.99	0.412
1F3B	HC	2.54	0.595
	MC	2.30	0.603
1F4B	HC	2.89	0.673
	MC	2.71	0.725

Abbreviations: HC = healthy children; MC = migraineur children; SD = standard deviation.

3.2. Multiple Flash Trials

We performed an ANOVA with three factors: (i) beep (two levels: 0 and 1), (ii) flash (three levels: 2-3-4), and (iii) group (two levels: healthy and migraineurs). The analysis showed the following results (Figures 3–5 and Table 3): the interaction flash for groups showed a main effect of F (2, 80) = 12.280, $p = 0.00002$; the factor group showed F (1, 40) = 14.608, $p = 0.00045$; in the factor beep, we found F (1, 40) = 59.940, $p = 0.00000$; in the factor flash, there was F (2, 80) = 186.97, $p = 0.00000$; in the interaction beep for groups, F (1, 40) = 1.7348, $p = 0.19530$; in the interaction beep for flash, F (2, 80) = 0.44831, $p = 0.64030$; in the interaction beep for flash for groups, F (2, 80) = 0.32853, $p = 0.72095$. The flash interaction of the groups' main effect is significant: F (2, 80) = 12.280, $p = 0.00002$. This indicates that the tendency to perceive a greater number of flashes in migraineurs increases with the number of flashes presented (without distinguishing between the presence or absence of beeps).

To highlight this difference, which represents the only significant difference between healthy children and migraineurs, we have also developed a measure for the perception of isolated flashes, expressed by the average value of flashes seen in all the conditions in which two or more flashes were presented without beeps (2F0B, 3F0B, 4F0B), which we defined as mean isolated flash perception (MIFP). The value of MIFP in migraineurs (2.89 ± 0.34) was significantly higher than in healthy children (2.31 ± 0.44), as determined using a t-test for unpaired data ($p = 0.0052$) (Figure 6).

Table 3. Multiple-flash trial results.

Test	Group	Mean	SD
2FB0	HC	2.06	0.447
	MC	2.25	0.380
2F1B	HC	1.57	0.562
	MC	1.93	0.403
3FB0	HC	2.38	0.470
	MC	2.87	0.407
3FB1	HC	1.95	0.670
	MC	2.60	0.465
4FB0	HC	2.67	0.575
	MC	3.33	0.429
4FB1	HC	2.23	0.662
	MC	2.96	0.522

Abbreviations: HC = healthy children; MC = migraineur children; SD = standard deviation.

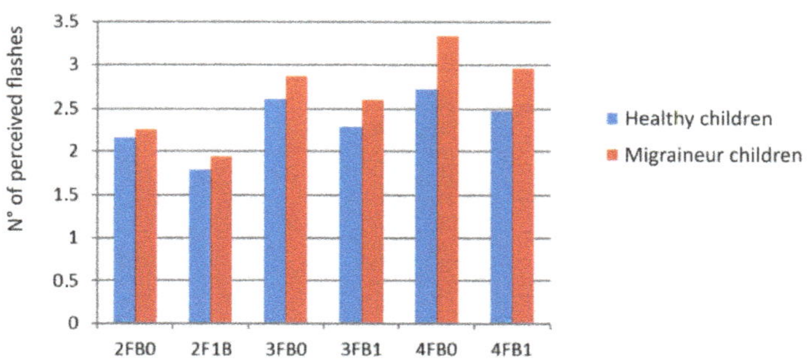

Figure 3. Fusion illusions in children with migraine and healthy children during multiple-flash trials. On the x-axis, the flashes (F) and beeps (B) combination of the different trials are given: for example, 1FB0 means the presentation of one flash and no beep. On the y-axis, the mean number of perceived flashes is reported.

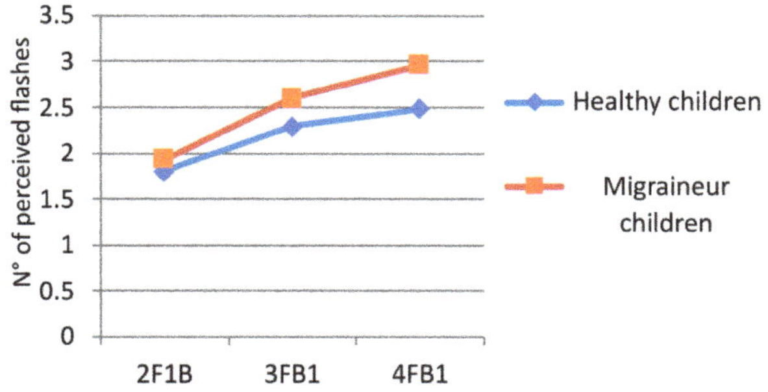

Figure 4. Flashes perceived with beeps during multiple-flash trials. On the x-axis, the flashes (F) and beeps (B) combination of the different trials are given: for example, 2F1B means the presentation of two flashes and one beep. On the y-axis, the mean number of perceived flashes is reported.

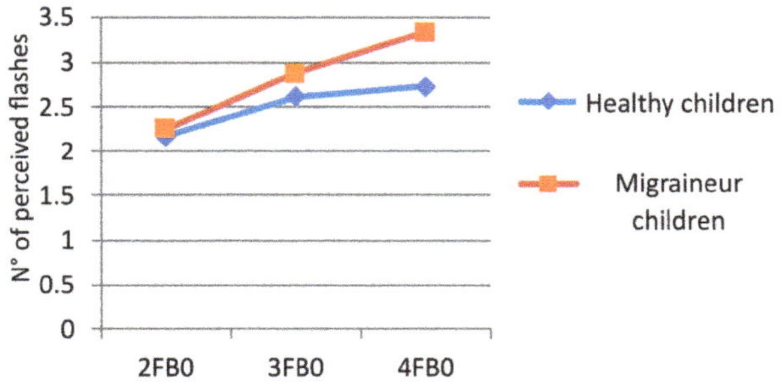

Figure 5. Flashes perceived without beeps during multiple-flash trials. On the x-axis, the flashes (F) and beeps (B) combination of the different trials are given: for example, 2FB0 means the presentation of two flashes and no beep. On the y-axis, the mean number of perceived flashes is reported.

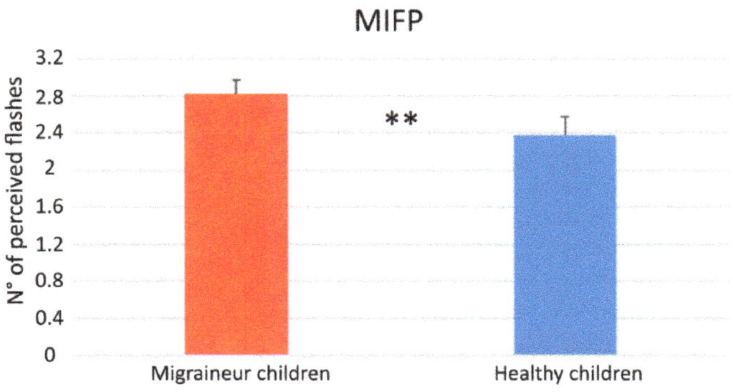

Figure 6. MIFP in children with migraine and healthy controls. MIFP: mean isolated flash perception. ** $p < 0.01$, using a *t*-test for unpaired data.

4. Discussion

In this study, we explored SIFIs in children affected by migraine without aura to evaluate if changes like those observed in adults in cross-modal illusory audio-visual phenomena could be found also in the developmental age. This was to evaluate a condition called visual cortical excitability, as seen in adults, and to explore potential changes due to evolving connections regarding cross-modal interaction in this age range.

Results from single-flash trials (i.e., used to evaluate the fission illusions) showed a slight, but not significant, reduction in fission illusions among migraineurs compared to healthy children regarding trial 1F3B. Differently, in multiple-flash trials (i.e., designed to explore the fusion illusions), patients perceived significantly more flashes than healthy subjects. This result, however, could not be attributed to a reduced fusion illusions phenomenon as it occurred in the combined (i.e., flash and beeps) and isolated flash trials, as shown by the specific MIFP measure elaborated to evaluate trials containing only isolated flashes (see results).

SIFIs depend on the cross-modal interaction of the acoustic and visual cortex and are specifically related to the excitability levels of these structures. It is, in fact, possible to experimentally interfere with this illusory perception using pre-conditioning with anodal or cathodal tDCS and by increasing the degree of responsiveness of the occipital cortex or reducing that of the temporal cortex, as demonstrated in healthy subjects by Bolognini et al. (2011) [26]. These data seem to indicate that the acoustic stimuli drive illusory visual perception: when these are reduced due to the inhibition of the acoustic cortex, or the transmission is less effective due to the increase in excitability of the visual cortex, the illusion disappears or fades. Brighina et al. observed a reduction in the illusory phenomenon in migraine patients that occurs both in the interictal phase (in migraineurs with aura) and during the attack (in patients with and without aura) [27]. This evidence fits well with the hypothesis of visual cortical hyperexcitability in migraine, which is present not only in the interictal condition (especially in patients with aura) but also during the attack when the lowest levels of fission illusions (i.e., highest cortical excitability) are reached. The result obtained by Brighina et al. (2015) underlines the importance of visual cortical hyperexcitability both in migraine with aura and without aura [27]. So, if hyperexcitability can represent the basis for triggering CSD in migraine with aura, it could well play a pathophysiological role in migraine without aura. This strengthens the hypothesis that, even in migraine with aura, a CSD-like mechanism called non-symptomatic CSD involving only silent cortical areas, even if not producing clinically appreciable aura phenomena, could still be capable of activating the trigeminal vascular system and triggering headache symptoms [32].

Neurophysiological investigations with different techniques have provided evidence about increased cortical excitability in adult migraineurs, underlining the importance not just of functional connectivity of cortical areas in the precipitation of the attack. Studies with TMS have shown an increase in cortical excitability (assessed by PT) in basic conditions or as a paradoxical response after rTMS at 1 Hz on the visual cortex compared to controls. An increase in excitability was also observed for visual associative areas responsible, for example, for the perception of moving images (i.e., V5 or motion-sensitive area MT), observing how the threshold for the induction of moving phosphenes—typically evoked by the stimulation of these areas—is reduced in migraineurs. Data in favor of greater cortical activation also come from studies performed with less subjective techniques compared to phosphenes, such as the magnetic suppression of perceptual accuracy (MPSA), which evaluates the interference induced by occipital magnetic stimulation on visual perceptual accuracy (percentage of recognition of groups of letters presented on a screen during occipital TMS) [33]. It is more difficult to generate interference effects on visual perception with occipital TMS in patients suffering from migraine with aura, and this effect is attributed to the lower efficiency of the inhibitory circuits [34,35].

Neurophysiological studies with visually evoked potentials conducted in migraineurs of developmental age have shown a greater amplitude of responses after visual stimulus compared to healthy subjects, confirming the abnormalities already found in adult migraineurs. Relevant insights regarding children with migraine also came about through the study of the recovery cycle of sensory-evoked potentials (i.e., a marker of cortical inhibitory efficiency) applied to evaluate the excitability of the somatosensory cortex. The results showed that the amplitude of the recovery cycle of cervical N13, N20, and P24 and cortical N30 was reduced compared to healthy controls, supporting the lower efficiency of cortical inhibition in migraineurs during childhood [36,37].

One of the objectives of our study was to investigate whether the hyperexcitability in migraine could modulate illusory perceptions in an immature multisensory integration system. The migraineurs' perception of fission illusions showed to be at the same level as healthy subjects, but from Figure 2, we can observe for the 1F3B combination, a minimal, albeit not significant, difference. Such results could suggest that the hyperexcitability of the occipital cortex requires a long time before it can emerge as it does in adult migraineurs because, when an individual is at an evolutionary age, the auditory dominance associated with multiple beeps interferes more with the determinism of the fission illusion. This indeed supports the data according to which the maturation of audio-visual integration systems occurs in conjunction with schooling [38]. As demonstrated by Nava et al. (2013), through sound-induced flash illusions, during growth, a transition occurs from auditory to visual sensory dominance in cross-modal perception processes [29].

However, it is not to be ruled out that the absence of a reduced number of fission illusions is due to the lack of opportunity to test subjects during the attack when greater visual cortical excitability is assumed [27]. In support of greater cortical excitability during an attack, Xiang et al. [37] demonstrated the presence of a dysfunction of the excitability of the motor cortex in migraine-suffering children through magnetoencephalography (MEG), where cerebral activation was elicited by finger tapping. The results showed a very high rate of activation of the cortex during the ictal phase and normalization during the interictal phase [38]. Other studies conducted with MEG and fMRI have confirmed that by inducing visual stress in patients with migraine, anomalous excitability of various cortical areas, such as the occipital, occipital-temporal, and occipital-parietal areas, is established, which is capable of triggering the aura or the attack, respectively, in migraineurs with or without aura [39,40].

However, from the analysis of multiple-flash trials, it emerged that even if migraineurs of developmental age do not perceive fewer illusions, they are able to perceive and discriminate multiple flashes better than controls of the same age ($p = 0.00002$). These data point out how children with migraine show an increased visual discrimination capacity even outside the attack. The visual system is relevant in migraine, as demonstrated for example by the symptom of photophobia, or by the role of cortical excitability and cortical activation (i.e., CSD) in aura determinism and migraine attacks. Further confirmations come from the neurophysiological studies with visual evoked potentials in children with migraine that showed a greater response after visual stimulation compared to healthy subjects [41]. Studies using TMS in the occipital cortex (with PT and suppression of visual perception) in migraine children without aura showed that migraineurs presented lower PTs than healthy participants at each time point, indicating increased occipital excitability. This was attenuated 1–2 days before a migraine attack, as indicated by a relative increase in PT. However, the increase in PTs before the next attack was associated with a stronger TMS-induced suppression of visual perception and a prolongation of the motion aftereffect. These findings show that pediatric migraine without aura is associated with a systematic shift in occipital excitability preceding the migraine attack [41–43].

Further suggestions come from this study, as by non-invasively studying the cortical excitability of children, it could be possible to monitor the efficacy of preventive therapies in patients with high-frequency migraine attacks. Supporting evidence comes from the study by Vollono et al. [44] in which improvement in the recovery cycle of somatosensory-evoked potential components with the use of topiramate was accompanied by an improvement in the frequency of migraine attacks. Conversely, subjects in whom this restoration of the cycle did not occur showed an ineffective response to topiramate. The authors concluded that their results suggest that topiramate efficacy was probably related to restored cortical excitability. The possibility of studying the efficacy of different pharmacological and non-pharmacological treatments in children at an early stage is also useful given parents' fear of the side effects of therapy. Further, cortical excitability in children with migraine seems to correlate with behavioral symptomatology [45].

In conclusion, we affirm the importance of multiple-flash trials to evaluate visual function in migraine during childhood. Even at an evolutionary age, there is already a remarkable hyper-responsiveness of the visual cortex, allowing us to say that probably the alterations of cortical excitability are already present at this age. Thus, the present study adds to the literature insight about a non-invasive marker of visual cortical function even in children with migraine.

This study, however, is still to be considered preliminary, and the following limitations are to be mentioned: it is necessary to conduct further experiments in the ictal phase to evaluate whether, similar to that which occurs in adults, the visual cortical excitability increases to oppose the illusory effect of acoustic stimulation during the audio-visual illusions. It is equally important to evaluate migraine children with aura in which a greater cortical excitability has been shown, or in pediatric chronic migraine where a more elevated cortical excitability was demonstrated compared to episodic migraine. Furthermore, the limited number of samples does not allow us to evaluate our results as a function of age, sex, frequency of attacks, and duration, which, in light of the above-mentioned considerations on the maturation process in children and variations in phenotype during developmental ages [2,3], are aspects that should not be overlooked. The absence in the control population of subjects suffering from tension-type headaches is an aspect that will need to be examined because at a developmental age, the boundaries between the two disorders are less clear than in adulthood, and there is frequently a transition from one form of headache to the other (more frequently from a tension-type headache to migraine) [46,47]. Finally, it would also be appropriate to compare our results with other non-invasive methods such as evoked potentials, quantitative EEG, etc., in the same subjects [48].

However, we believe that this study can help generate new hypotheses for research using non-invasive methods, and clinically, supported by other studies, SIFIs could represent an early marker of cortex hyper-responsiveness to identify pediatric migraine.

Author Contributions: Conceptualization F.B.; Methodology S.D.M., F.B., L.P., G.C., B.F. and V.R.; Software S.M. and A.S.; Validation V.R.; Formal analysis S.D.M., L.P., F.B. and V.R.; Investigation S.D.M., L.P. and S.M.; Resources E.C., A.S. and L.P.; Data curation S.M., E.C., F.B., S.D.M., A.S. and V.R.; Writing—original draft, S.D.M., L.P., B.F., V.R. and F.B.; Writing—review and editing L.P., S.D.M., B.F, V.R. and A.T.; Supervision V.R., B.F. and F.B. All authors have read and agreed to the published version of the manuscript.

Funding: The medical writing was funded through a donation from Allergan S.p.A., Italy with the approval n. 1318/2021 of 20 December 2021.

Institutional Review Board Statement: The study was approved by the Palermo 1 Ethics Committee (Palermo, Italy). The protocol number is no. 5/2015 of 13 May 2015.

Informed Consent Statement: An informed consent was obtained from "the parents" of all subjects involved in the study.

Data Availability Statement: Data are available upon reasonable request to the corresponding author. The data are not publicly available due to privacy restrictions.

Conflicts of Interest: The authors declare that this study received funding from Allergan S.p.A., Italy. The funder was not involved in the study design, collection, analysis, interpretation of data, the writing of this article or the decision to submit it for publication.

References

1. Onofri, A.; Pensato, U.; Rosignoli, C.; Wells-Gatnik, W.; Stanyer, E.; Ornello, R.; Chen, H.Z.; De Santis, F.; Torrente, A.; Mikulenka, P.; et al. Primary headache epidemiology in children and adolescents: A systematic review and meta-analysis. *J. Headache Pain* **2023**, *24*, 8. [CrossRef] [PubMed]
2. Lewis, D.W. Pediatric migraine. *Pediatr. Rev.* **2007**, *28*, 43–53. [CrossRef] [PubMed]
3. Raieli, V.; D'Amico, A.; Piro, E. Migraine in Children Under 7 Years of Age: A Review. *Curr. Pain Headache Rep.* **2020**, *24*, 79. [CrossRef] [PubMed]
4. García-Azorín, D.; Moya-Alarcón, C.; Armada, B.; Sánchez del Río, M. Societal and economic burden of migraine in Spain: Results from the 2020 National Health and Wellness Survey. *J. Headache Pain* **2024**, *25*, 38. [CrossRef] [PubMed]

5. Mazzotta, G.; Gallai, B.; Mattioni, A.; Floridi, F.; Foti, F.; Allegretti, M.; D'angelo, R. Cost assessment of headache in childhood and adolescence: Preliminary data. *J. Headache Pain* **2005**, *6*, 281–283. [CrossRef] [PubMed]
6. Finning, K.; Neochoriti Varvarrigou, I.; Ford, T.; Panagi, L.; Ukoumunne, O.C. Mental health and school absenteeism in children with long-term physical conditions: A secondary analysis of the British Child and Adolescent Mental Health Surveys 2004 and 2007. *Child Care Health Dev.* **2022**, *48*, 110–119. [CrossRef] [PubMed]
7. Dodick, D.W. A Phase-by-Phase Review of Migraine Pathophysiology. *Headache* **2018**, *58*, 4–16. [CrossRef] [PubMed]
8. Olesen, J. Headache Classification Committee of the International Headache Society (IHS) The International Classification of Headache Disorders, 3rd edition. *Cephalalgia* **2018**, *38*, 1–211.
9. Bose, P.; Karsan, N.; Goadsby, P.J. The Migraine Postdrome. *Contin. Lifelong Learn. Neurol.* **2018**, *24*, 1023–1031. [CrossRef]
10. Gelfand, A.A.; Goadsby, P.J.; Allen, I.E. The relationship between migraine and infant colic: A systematic review and meta-analysis. *Cephalalgia* **2015**, *35*, 63–72. [CrossRef]
11. Özge, A.; Abu-Arafeh, I.; Gelfand, A.A.; Goadsby, P.J.; Cuvellier, J.C.; Valeriani, M.; Sergeev, A.; Barlow, K.; Uludüz, D.; Yalın, O.; et al. Experts' opinion about the pediatric secondary headaches diagnostic criteria of the ICHD-3 beta. *J. Headache Pain* **2017**, *18*, 113. [CrossRef] [PubMed]
12. Raieli, V.; Capizzi, M.; Marino, A.; Di Nardo, G.; Raucci, U.; Parisi, P. Study on "Atypical" Migraine Auras in the Pediatric Age: The Role of Cortical Spreading Depression and the Physiopathogenetic Hypothesis Arising from Our Clinical Cases. *Life* **2022**, *12*, 450. [CrossRef] [PubMed]
13. Gelfand, A.A.; Reider, A.C.; Goadsby, P.J. Cranial autonomic symptoms in pediatric migraine are the rule, not the exception. *Neurology* **2013**, *81*, 431–436. [CrossRef] [PubMed]
14. Jernigan, T.L.; Baaré, W.F.C.; Stiles, J.; Madsen, K.S. Postnatal brain development: Structural imaging of dynamic neurodevelopmental processes. *Prog. Brain Res.* **2011**, *189*, 77–92. [PubMed]
15. Stiles, J.; Jernigan, T.L. The basics of brain development. *Neuropsychol. Rev.* **2010**, *20*, 327–348. [CrossRef] [PubMed]
16. Guidetti, V.; Galli, F.; Termine, C. Headache in children. *Handb. Clin. Neurol.* **2010**, *97*, 739–754. [PubMed]
17. Deodato, M.; Granato, A.; Martini, M.; Stella, A.B.; Galmonte, A.; Murena, L.; Manganotti, P. Neurophysiological and Clinical Outcomes in Episodic Migraine without Aura: A Cross-Sectional Study. *J. Clin. Neurophysiol.* **2024**. [CrossRef]
18. Goadsby, P.J.; Holland, P.R.; Martins-Oliveira, M.; Hoffmann, J.; Schankin, C.; Akerman, S. Pathophysiology of Migraine: A Disorder of Sensory Processing. *Physiol. Rev.* **2017**, *97*, 553–622. [CrossRef] [PubMed]
19. Dichgans, M.; Freilinger, T.; Eckstein, G.; Babini, E.; Lorenz-Depiereux, B.; Biskup, S.; Ferrari, M.D.; Herzog, J.; van den Maagdenberg, A.M.J.M.; Pusch, M.; et al. Mutation in the neuronal voltage-gated sodium channel SCN1A in familial hemiplegic migraine. *Lancet* **2005**, *366*, 371–377. [CrossRef]
20. Van den Maagdenberg, A.M.; Pietrobon, D.; Pizzorusso, T.; Kaja, S.; Broos, L.A.; Cesetti, T.; van de Ven, R.C.; Tottene, A.; van der Kaa, J.; Plomp, J.J.; et al. A Cacna1a knockin migraine mouse model with increased susceptibility to cortical spreading depression. *Neuron* **2004**, *41*, 701–710. [CrossRef]
21. Ophoff, R.A.; Terwindt, G.M.; Vergouwe, M.N.; van Eijk, R.; Oefner, P.J.; Hoffman, S.M.; Lamerdin, J.E.; Mohrenweiser, H.W.; Bulman, D.E.; Ferrari, M.; et al. Familial hemiplegic migraine and episodic ataxia type-2 are caused by mutations in the Ca^{2+} channel gene CACNL1A4. *Cell* **1996**, *87*, 543–552. [CrossRef] [PubMed]
22. Creutzfeldt, O.D.; Fromm, G.H.; Kapp, H. Influence of transcortical d-c currents on cortical neuronal activity. *Exp. Neurol.* **1962**, *5*, 436–452. [CrossRef] [PubMed]
23. Cosentino, G.; Di Marco, S.; Ferlisi, S.; Valentino, F.; Capitano, W.M.; Fierro, B.; Brighina, F. Intracortical facilitation within the migraine motor cortex depends on the stimulation intensity. A paired-pulse TMS study. *J. Headache Pain* **2018**, *19*, 65. [CrossRef] [PubMed]
24. Brighina, F.; Piazza, A.; Daniele, O.; Fierro, B. Modulation of visual cortical excitability in migraine with aura: Effects of 1 Hz repetitive transcranial magnetic stimulation. *Exp. Brain Res.* **2002**, *145*, 177–181. [CrossRef] [PubMed]
25. Shams, L.; Kamitani, Y.; Shimojo, S. What you see is what you hear. *Nature* **2000**, *408*, 788. [CrossRef] [PubMed]
26. Bolognini, N.; Rossetti, A.; Casati, C.; Mancini, F.; Vallar, G. Neuromodulation of multisensory perception: A tDCS study of the sound-induced flash illusion. *Neuropsychologia* **2011**, *49*, 231–237. [CrossRef] [PubMed]
27. Brighina, F.; Bolognini, N.; Cosentino, G.; Maccora, S.; Paladino, P.; Baschi, R.; Vallar, G.; Fierro, B. Visual cortex hyperexcitability in migraine in response to sound-induced flash illusions. *Neurology* **2015**, *84*, 2057–2061. [CrossRef] [PubMed]
28. Innes-Brown, H.; Barutchu, A.; Shivdasani, M.N.; Crewther, D.P.; Grayden, D.B.; Paolini, A.G. Susceptibility to the flash-beep illusion is increased in children compared to adults. *Dev. Sci.* **2011**, *14*, 1089–1099. [CrossRef] [PubMed]
29. Nava, E.; Pavani, F. Changes in sensory dominance during childhood: Converging evidence from the colavita effect and the sound-induced flash illusion. *Child. Dev.* **2013**, *84*, 604–616. [CrossRef]
30. Afra, J.; Mascia, A.; Gérard, P.; Maertens de Noordhout, A.; Schoenen, J. Interictal cortical excitability in migraine: A study using transcranial magnetic stimulation of motor and visual cortices. *Ann. Neurol.* **1998**, *44*, 209–215. [CrossRef]
31. Headache Classification Committee of the International Headache Society (IHS). The International Classification of Headache Disorders, 3rd edition (beta version). *Cephalalgia* **2013**, *33*, 629–808. [CrossRef]
32. Zhang, X.; Levy, D.; Kainz, V.; Noseda, R.; Jakubowski, M.; Burstein, R. Activation of central trigeminovascular neurons by cortical spreading depression. *Ann. Neurol.* **2011**, *69*, 855–865. [CrossRef]

33. Mulleners, W.M.; Chronicle, E.P.; Palmer, J.E.; Koehler, P.J.; Vredeveld, J.W. Visual cortex excitability in migraine with and without aura. *Headache* **2001**, *41*, 565–572. [CrossRef] [PubMed]
34. Battelli, L.; Black, K.R.; Wray, S.H. Transcranial magnetic stimulation of visual area V5 in migraine. *Neurology* **2002**, *58*, 1066–1069. [CrossRef] [PubMed]
35. Custers, A.; Mulleners, W.M.; Chronicle, E.P. Assessing cortical excitability in migraine: Reliability of magnetic suppression of perceptual accuracy technique over time. *Headache* **2005**, *45*, 1202–1207. [CrossRef] [PubMed]
36. Pro, S.; Tarantino, S.; Capuano, A.; Vigevano, F.; Valeriani, M. Primary headache pathophysiology in children: The contribution of clinical neurophysiology. *Clin. Neurophysiol.* **2014**, *125*, 6–12. [CrossRef] [PubMed]
37. Xiang, J.; Degrauw, X.; Korostenskaja, M.; Korman, A.M.; O'Brien, H.L.; Kabbouche, M.A.; Powers, S.W.; Hershey, A.D. Altered cortical activation in adolescents with acute migraine: A magnetoencephalography study. *J. Pain* **2013**, *14*, 1553–1563. [CrossRef]
38. Leiken, K.A.; Xiang, J.; Curry, E.; Fujiwara, H.; Rose, D.F.; Allen, J.R.; Kacperski, J.E.; O'brien, H.L.; Kabbouche, M.A.; Powers, S.W.; et al. Quantitative neuromagnetic signatures of aberrant cortical excitability in pediatric chronic migraine. *J. Headache Pain* **2016**, *17*, 46. [CrossRef] [PubMed]
39. Bowyer, S.M.; Aurora, K.S.; Moran, J.E.; Tepley, N.; Welch, K.M. Magnetoencephalographic fields from patients with spontaneous and induced migraine aura. *Ann. Neurol.* **2001**, *50*, 582–587. [CrossRef]
40. Cao, Y.; Welch, K.M.; Aurora, S.; Vikingstad, E.M. Functional MRI-BOLD of visually triggered headache in patients with migraine. *Arch. Neurol.* **1999**, *56*, 548–554. [CrossRef]
41. Akin, O.; Ünay, B.; Arslan, M.; Mazman, S.; Taşçilar, E.; Eker, I. Evaluation of somatosensory evoked potentials (SEPs) in obese children. *Gulhane Med. J.* **2018**, *60*, 5–8. [CrossRef]
42. Ernst, M.O. Multisensory integration: A late bloomer. *Curr. Biol.* **2008**, *18*, R519–R521. [CrossRef] [PubMed]
43. Siniatchkin, M.; Reich, A.L.; Shepherd, A.J.; van Baalen, A.; Siebner, H.R.; Stephani, U. Peri-ictal changes of cortical excitability in children suffering from migraine without aura. *Pain* **2009**, *147*, 132–140. [CrossRef] [PubMed]
44. Vollono, C.; Ferraro, D.; Miliucci, R.; Vigevano, F.; Valeriani, M. The abnormal recovery cycle of somatosensory evoked potential components in children with migraine can be reversed by topiramate. *Cephalalgia* **2010**, *30*, 17–26. [CrossRef] [PubMed]
45. Valeriani, M.; Galli, F.; Tarantino, S.; Graceffa, D.; Pignata, E.; Miliucci, R.; Biondi, G.; Tozzi, A.; Vigevano, F.; Guidetti, V. Correlation between abnormal brain excitability and emotional symptomatology in paediatric migraine. *Cephalalgia* **2009**, *29*, 204–213. [CrossRef] [PubMed]
46. Baglioni, V.; Orecchio, S.; Esposito, D.; Faedda, N.; Natalucci, G.; Guidetti, V. Tension-Type Headache in Children and Adolescents. *Life* **2023**, *13*, 825. [CrossRef] [PubMed]
47. Onan, D.; Younis, S.; Wellsgatnik, W.D.; Farham, F.; Andruškevičius, S.; Abashidze, A.; Jusupova, A.; Romanenko, Y.; Grosu, O.; Moldokulova, M.Z.; et al. Debate: Differences and similarities between tension-type headache and migraine. *J. Headache Pain* **2023**, *24*, 92. [CrossRef]
48. Puca, F.; de Tommaso, M. Clinical neurophysiology in childhood headache. *Cephalalgia* **1999**, *19*, 137–146. [CrossRef]

children

MDPI

Article

The Photo- and Phonosensitivity Avoidance Behavior Scales: Evaluating Clinical Utility in Pediatric Primary Chronic Headache

Allison M. Smith [1,2,*], Megan N. Silvia [3], Hannah Rogan [1] and Alyssa A. Lebel [1,4]

1 Division of Pain Medicine, Department of Anesthesiology, Perioperative and Pain Medicine, Boston Children's Hospital, Boston, MA 02215, USA; hannah.rogan@childrens.harvard.edu (H.R.); alyssa.lebel@childrens.harvard.edu (A.A.L.)

2 Division of Psychology, Department of Psychiatry, Harvard Medical School, Boston, MA 02215, USA

3 School of Occupational Therapy, Massachusetts College of Pharmacy & Health Sciences, Boston, MA 02215, USA; megan.silvia@mcphs.edu

4 Department of Anesthesia, Harvard Medical School, Boston, MA 02215, USA

* Correspondence: allison.smith@childrens.harvard.edu; Tel.: +1-781-216-1960

Abstract: Background/Objectives: Pediatric primary chronic headache disorders are often associated with sensitivities to light (photosensitivity) and sound (phonosensitivity) that may trigger or worsen headache pain. These sensory sensitivities may result in changes to activity participation or environmental modifications to avoid visual and auditory stimuli. Over time, avoidance behaviors can inadvertently increase functional disability, suggesting the importance of their thorough consideration. The PhotoSensitivity and PhonoSensitivity Avoidance Behavior Scales (PHOTO-SABS and PHONO-SABS, respectively) were recently developed and preliminarily validated to assist clinicians in evaluating such behaviors. This study aimed to confirm each of their factor structures in a new sample and enhance their clinical utility. **Methods**: A sample of 176 youth (aged 8–17) with a primary chronic headache diagnosis completed the PHOTO-SABS and PHONO-SABS as part of their multidisciplinary evaluation in a pediatric headache clinic. **Results**: Consistent with the previous validation, confirmatory factor analyses supported a two-factor model for the PHOTO-SABS and a single-factor model for the PHONO-SABS. Tertile groupings (low, moderate, high) provided the most appropriate clinical reference points. The relative change criterion (RCCrit) was established at 6.4 points for both measures. **Conclusions**: These findings confirm that the PHOTO- and PHONO-SABS are psychometrically robust tools for clinicians to evaluate sensitivity-related avoidance behavior and to monitor response to interventions in youth with primary chronic headaches.

Keywords: primary chronic headache; chronic pain; phonosensitivity; avoidance

1. Introduction

A 2024 systematic review and meta-analysis [1] indicated that the overall prevalence of chronic headaches (headaches persisting more than three months) in children and adolescents is remarkably high, at 25.7%, across chronic migraine with/without aura, chronic tension-type headaches, New Daily Persistent Headache (NDPH), and other chronic headache subtypes. In addition to the discomfort itself, chronic headaches in youth are responsible for considerable comorbid functional disability, reflected in impairment across physical, social, emotional, and academic domains [2–4]. Given the extensive economic burden, comorbidities, and impact on quality of life associated with chronic headaches [5–7], the ability to understand and accurately assess factors contributing to headache-related disability represents an important area of research.

When examining pediatric chronic headache, it is critical to examine not only the severity and impact of head pain itself but also those of its associated features, as these too can contribute to severe functional impairment and poorer quality of life [8,9]. One subset of associated features worth noting, considering the central nervous system's role in chronic headache and chronic pain [10,11] and the potential for impact on functioning, is heightened sensitivity to non-noxious sensory stimuli (e.g., visual, auditory, olfactory, somatosensory) [12]. Though migraine is most often associated with these hypersensitivities (e.g., photophobia, phonophobia, osmophobia), more recent explorations of headache subtypes in children and adolescents reveal that such sensory sensitivities are present across pediatric chronic headache presentations. For instance, when comparing youth diagnosed with chronic migraine with/without aura, chronic tension-type headache, and NDPH, Reidy et al. (2020) [8] identified no clinically meaningful differences in associated features, including photophobia and phonophobia, or in degree of functional disability. Similarly, Strong et al. (2021) [13] reported that the overwhelming majority (85%) of pediatric patients with NDPH experience photophobia and/or phonophobia, as well as reduced activity levels (88%).

Historically, to explain the relationship between the experience of chronic pain and functional disability, researchers have turned to the Fear-Avoidance Model (FAM) [14]. This model emphasizes that pain-related catastrophizing, fear, and avoidance behavior are critical contributors to the cycle of pain-related disability. When an individual perceives a pain-associated stimulus as a threat, they may come to fear the stimulus and pain; such fears can precipitate avoidance. Thus, one may become increasingly disabled as attempts to avoid pain and its related stimuli generalize. In fact, in their pediatric application of the FAM, Simons and Kaczynski (2012) [15] noted that avoidance behavior is a "more proximal link to functional outcomes", as compared to pain-related fear or pain catastrophizing, likely due to its behavioral nature.

The FAM can be applied to the relationship between the associated headache features of light/sound sensitivities and headache-related disability, as avoidance of sensory input predicts functional disability in youth with headached [9]. However, despite this understanding (i.e., that headache-related sensory sensitivities are relevant across subtypes and that their avoidance contributes to disability), until recently, there were no validated measures of avoidance behavior specifically in youth with chronic headaches. Over a decade ago, Simons and colleagues (2011) [16] validated the Fear of Pain Questionnaire—Child Report (FOPQ-C), a standardized, commonly used tool for assessing pain-related fear and avoidance in youth with chronic pain. When analyzing their findings by pain subgroup [17], the authors noted that numerous FOPQ-C items are based upon fear/avoidance of movement, rendering them less relevant to patients with chronic headaches, as compared to potential items about cognitive demand or sensory input.

Further, in the literature, often, either fear and avoidance are examined in parallel (i.e., within the same measure) or fear is utilized as a proxy for avoidance. However, some researchers [18] highlight that fear and avoidance are related but not synonymous constructs. In fact, given that excessive avoidance behavior most directly contributes to pain-related disability and deleterious outcomes, avoidance behavior should thus be examined separately from fear.

To address the gap in the literature on avoidance behavior related to sensory sensitivities in pediatric chronic headaches, our group recently developed [19] and provided initial validation [20] of the PhotoSensitivity Avoidance Behavior Scale (PHOTO-SABS) and PhonoSensitivity Avoidance Behavior Scale (PHONO-SABS). The first phase was multistep measure development, whereby an expert panel generated relevant items and then a pilot sample was employed to establish the measures' feasibility and understandability for completion. This entailed measure administration followed by cognitive interviews [19]. In the second phase, the measures were improved and empirically validated in a large, new sample, exploring individual item performance, factor structure, internal consistency, and item content. Both measures demonstrated strong internal consistency, construct validity, and criterion-related validity [20]. At present, both measures have been integrated successfully into outpatient clinics and intensive pain rehabilitation settings. However, there has not yet been replication to confirm the measures' factor structures, nor has there been specific consideration of the measures' clinical utility.

Thus, the purpose of this final phase was two-fold: (1) to confirm the factor structures of the PHOTO- and PHONO-SABS, and (2) to increase their clinical utility by delineating clinical reference points and the reliable change criteria (RCCrit) for each measure. This would finalize psychometrically sound tools for health care clinicians to evaluate functioning and measure response to intervention in youth with primary chronic headaches.

2. Materials and Methods

2.1. Participants

Youth ($N = 176$) aged 8–17 who sought initial evaluation at a multidisciplinary chronic headache program between May 2022 and May 2023 at an urban, pediatric hospital in the U.S. participated in the study. Much of the sample described their race as White, their sex assigned at birth as "female", and their gender identity as "cisgender female". These demographics are generally representative of the population of youth typically presenting to this tertiary clinic. See Table 1 below for more detailed demographic information.

Table 1. Self-reported demographic and headache history variables.

	N	%	Mean	SD
Age			14.73	2.45
Sex Assigned at Birth				
Female	132	75		
Male	44	25		
Gender Identity				
Cisgender Female	127	72.2		
Cisgender Male	43	24.4		
Non-Binary	2	1.1		
Transgender	1	0.6		
Not Reported	3	1.7		
Race				
White	134	76.2		
Black or African American	3	1.7		
Asian American	2	1.1		
Multiracial	4	2.3		
Not Reported	12	18.7		
Ethnicity				
Non-Hispanic	145	89.2		
Hispanic	19	10.8		
Chronic Headache (HA) Diagnosis				
Chronic Migraine (CM)	69	39.2		
New Daily Persistent Headache (NDPH)	41	23.3		
Mixed Type (CM with CTTH)	39	22.2		
Chronic Tension-Type Headache (CTTH)	19	10.8		
Diagnosis unavailable	8	4.5		
Chronic Headache Presentation				
Time Since Onset (Months)			42.9	62.75
Typical Pain Intensity Rating (NRS)			7.34	1.82
Frequency = Daily/Constant	89	50.6		

Physician-assigned chronic headache diagnoses were based upon the International Headache Society's International Classification of Headache Disorders, third editions (ICHD-3 [21]). Only patients with primary chronic headaches were included; patients with acute headache presentations or headaches secondary to another general medical condition were not included. Most participants had been coping with headaches for several years, with more than half reporting daily/constant headache.

Participant diagnoses included the following: chronic Migraine with/without aura (1.3 in the ICHD-3), Intractable/Chronic Tension-Type Headache (2.3 in the ICHD-3 [22]), and/or New Daily Persistent Headache (4.10 in the ICHD-3). There was also a notable subgroup of patients meeting criteria for chronic migraine who also met criteria for Intractable/Chronic Tension-Type Headache (often referred to clinically as "mixed" type [23]). While the latter is not an explicit ICHD-3 headache diagnosis, in pediatrics, chronic migraine and chronic tension-type headaches often co-exist and "may represent a distinct headache type" [23], which may also influence how youth with this presentation experience associated symptoms and respond to intervention.

2.2. Measures

2.2.1. Pain Severity

The Numeric Rating Scale (NRS) [24] was utilized to evaluate pain intensity. Participants were asked to designate their typical pain level on a standard 11-point scale, ranging from 0 (indicating "no pain") to 10 (indicating "the most pain imaginable").

2.2.2. Pain-Related Fear & Avoidance Behavior

The PhotoSensitivity Avoidance Behavior Scale (PHOTO-SABS) [20] is an 11-item self-report tool that evaluates behavioral responses to headache-related photosensitivity (i.e., perceived sensitivity to light). Each item asks participants to respond on a four-point Likert-type scale, ranging from "Never" to "Always", with higher ratings reflecting greater avoidance or modification of the environment to accommodate photosensitivity. The PHOTO-SABS demonstrated a Cronbach's alpha of 0.92 in the initial validation study, which also revealed two correlated but distinct subscales: challenges to participation and modification of environment.

The PhonoSensitivity Avoidance Behavior Scale (PHONO-SABS) [20] is a 12-item self-report tool that evaluates behavioral responses to headache-related phonosensitivity (i.e., perceived sensitivity to sound). Each item asks participants to respond on a four-point Likert-type scale, ranging from "Never" to "Always", with higher ratings reflecting greater avoidance or modification of the environment to accommodate phonosensitivity. The PHONO-SABS demonstrated a Cronbach's alpha of 0.92 in the initial validation study, which revealed a single scale for the measure (i.e., no subscales).

The Fear of Pain Questionnaire—Child report (FOPQ-C) [16] is a self-report inventory that assesses pain-related fear and associated avoidance behaviors in youth. Participants respond on a five-point Likert-type scale, ranging from "Strongly Disagree" to "Strongly Agree". A total score is derived by summing the ratings, with higher scores indicating greater fear and avoidance related to pain. There are also two validated subscales, fear of pain and avoidance of activities, both of which were examined in this study.

2.2.3. Headache-Related Impairment

The Headache Impact Test (HIT-6) [25,26] assesses youth perception of the specific impact of headache on daily life over the course of four weeks. Its six items evaluate the adverse impact of headache on various aspects of functioning, as well as the severity of headache pain. Participants respond using a five-point Likert-type scale, ranging from "Never" to "Always". A total score is derived from the sum of the ratings, with higher scores reflecting a greater impact of headache pain on daily life.

The SChool REfusal EvaluatioN (SCREEN) [27] is an 18-item self-report tool designed to assess school avoidance and refusal in children and adolescents. Responses are scored on a five-point Likert-type scale, ranging from "Doesn't apply to me at all" to "Applies to me completely". Ratings can be summed to calculate a total score that can then be categorized by clinical reference points. There are in four subscales as well: Anxious Anticipation, Difficult Transition, Interpersonal Discomfort, and School Avoidance. The SCREEN School Avoidance (SCREEN-SA) subscale score was used in this study. Higher scores reflect greater school avoidance.

Pediatric Migraine Disability Assessment (PedMIDAS) [28] is a self-report inventory consisting of six-items that evaluate the impact of headache across several domains (e.g., school functioning, activities within the home, activities outside of the home). Participants indicate the number of days in the past three months that their functioning was affected by headaches. For the purposes of this study, the two items pertaining to functioning at home and functioning in activities outside of the home were examined at the individual level. Higher scores reflect a greater impact of headache on functioning.

2.3. Procedure

Before their initial multidisciplinary evaluation in the chronic headache program, youth and their caregivers are requested to complete standardized surveys through a secure electronic platform as a standard component of routine clinical care. These surveys gather information on pain, developmental and medical history, and psychological functioning. These clinical data are kept in a centralized data repository, the Chronic Pain Data Repository, which stores patient data for those treated in all of the institution's pain-related clinical settings [29]. The repository has been overseen by an ongoing standardized research protocol approved by the hospital's institutional review board (IRB) since October 2018. Researchers can formally apply to access de-identified data, by providing a data safety and monitoring plan, obtaining approval of the departmental scientific review committee, and signing a data use agreement. Importantly, while patients and families are strongly encouraged to complete these standardized surveys prior to their visit, their completion is not mandatory. Patients received all medically indicated treatments regardless of whether they completed the surveys.

2.4. Statistical Analyses

Data were analyzed with SPSS version 29 and SPSS-AMOS version 26. Descriptive statistics were performed to assess underlying assumptions of normality for all variables. To confirm the factor structures of the two original measures, the PHOTO-SABS and the PHONO-SABS, we performed a series of Confirmatory Factor Analyses. For the PHOTO-SABS, we also examined whether one factor was more parsimonious than the original two-factor structure. As the PHONO-SABS was originally determined to have a single factor, additional models were unnecessary. Goodness of model fit for each measure was assessed using a chi-square significance test (χ^2), as well as the following indices of fit: χ^2/df (<3.0 good, <5.0 acceptable), comparative fit index (CFI; >0.90 acceptable, >0.95 excellent), and root mean square error of approximation (RMSEA; <0.08 acceptable, <0.05 excellent) using their agreed upon benchmarks [30,31].

Based upon methods previously utilized to determine clinical reference points for similar measures pertaining to pediatric pain [32–34], we examined tertile and quartile groupings of PHOTO-SABS and PHONO-SABS scores. We sought to identify the most parsimonious classification systems for the PHOTO-SABS and the PHONO-SABS that aligned with statistically significant differences in pain-related fear and avoidance, headache-related impact on life, and school/activity functioning. These groupings would reflect distinct and clinically meaningful reference points for both measures. We followed the same procedure for each measure, so the process is described here once. We first classified PHOTO-SABS scores into three levels (i.e., low, moderate, high), using tertile groups based on score distributions. We then conducted a series of one-tailed, one-way ANOVAs with Tukey post hoc analyses to confirm the validity of the tertile classification system. To confirm that tertile reference points were clinically meaningful, we sought significant group differences in selected measures of construct and criterion validity. We examined the Tukey post hoc analyses, applying a Bonferroni correction for multiple analyses ($p < 0.007$) to account for potential inflation of the Type I error rate. Finally, to ensure that tertiles were indeed the most parsimonious grouping option, we re-classified PHOTO-SABS scores into four levels (i.e., none/minimal, low, moderate, high), using quartile groupings based on score distributions, repeating the process. We followed the same steps to determine clinical reference points for PHONO-SABS scores.

Finally, we calculated the reliable change criterion (RCCrit) to aid in evaluating potential changes in photo- and phonosensitivity avoidance behavior over time (e.g., before and after intervention). Following the procedure standardized in previous studies of similar measures [33,35], we calculated RCCrit from the standard deviation (*SD*) and the measure's reliability estimate (i.e., Cronbach's alpha, *rel*), using the following formula: RCCrit = $(SD \times \sqrt{2} \times \sqrt{1 - rel}) \times 1.96$. The RCCrits established here for the PHOTO-SABS and PHONO-SABS can be used to determine whether changes in photo- and phonosensitivity-related avoidance behavior scores are due to true changes (i.e., treatment response) or due to measurement error.

3. Results

3.1. Confirmatory Factor Analysis: PHOTO-SABS

The PHOTO-SABS items were analyzed to confirm their contributions to the scale. None of the 11 items violated assumptions of normality (i.e., skew and kurtosis for all items were <2.0). Participant responses spanned the possible range (0–3) for all items. The CFA with items constrained to their original two-factor structure yielded a nearly acceptable model fit, though modification indices revealed covariance in the error terms that needed to be accounted for. Upon re-running the CFA with the same set of items, and with error covariances accounted for, the model demonstrated acceptable to excellent fit ($\chi^2 = 84.13$, $p < 0.001$, $\chi^2/df = 2.16$, CFI = 0.96, and RMSEA = 0.08). Figure 1 shows the final model with standardized regression coefficients/factor loadings (β) for the PHOTO-SABS subscales, which were strong, ranging from β = 0.54 to 0.88. By comparison, the single-factor model of the PHOTO-SABS showed a poor fit, confirming the necessity of including both factors. The PHOTO-SABS total score had a Cronbach's α of 0.91, with a sample mean of 11.49 (SD = 7.72). The two subscales were each internally consistent (Changes to Participation α = 0.89, Modification of Environment α = 0.83) and intercorrelated, yet distinct ($r = 0.69$, $p < 0.001$). Total and subscale scores were normally distributed across the sample.

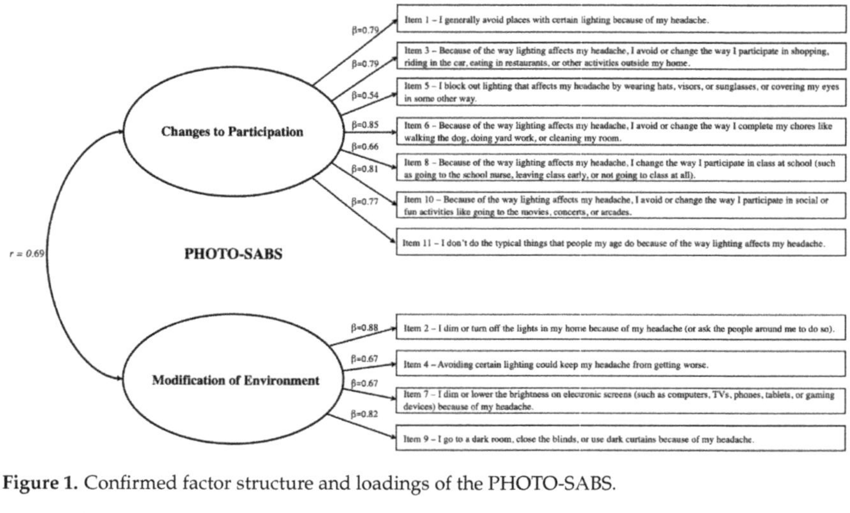

Figure 1. Confirmed factor structure and loadings of the PHOTO-SABS.

3.2. Confirmatory Factor Analysis: PHONO-SABS

In the same manner, the 12 PHONO-SABS items were analyzed to confirm their contributions to the scale. No items violated assumptions of normality (i.e., skew and kurtosis for all items were >2.0). Again, all participant responses spanned the possible range (0–3). The CFA, with items constrained to their original single-factor structure, initially yielded a nearly acceptable model fit, though once again, modification indices revealed covariance in the error terms that needed to be accounted for. Upon re-running the CFA with the same items, and with error covariances accounted for, the updated PHONO-SABS model demonstrated acceptable to excellent fit ($\chi^2 = 116.60$, $p < 0.001$, $\chi^2/df = 2.33$, CFI = 0.95, and RMSEA = 0.08). Figure 2 shows the final model with standardized regression coefficients/factor loadings (β) for the PHONO-SABS, which were strong, ranging from β = 0.55 to 0.88. The PHONO-SABS total score had a Cronbach's α of 0.93, with a sample mean of 10.77 (SD = 8.78). Total scores were normally distributed across the sample.

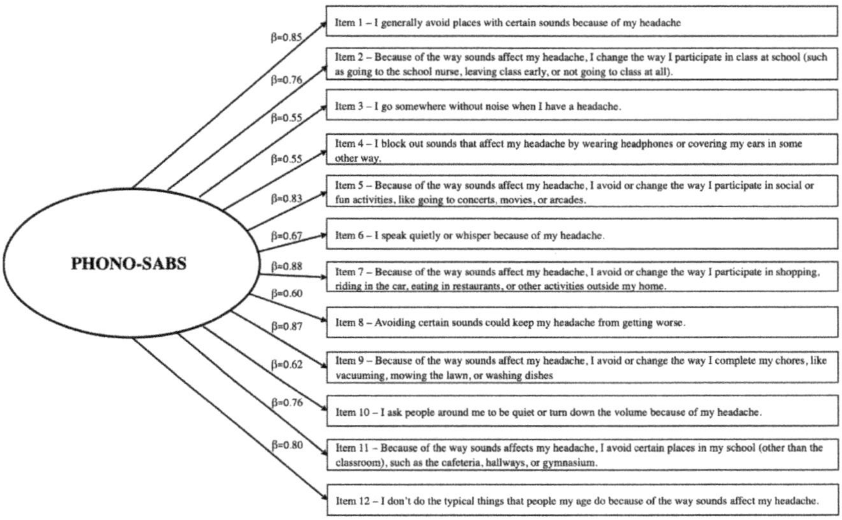

Figure 2. Confirmed factor structure and loadings of the PHONO-SABS.

3.3. Clinical Reference Points: PHOTO-SABS

PHOTO-SABS scores in the lowest tertile (i.e., scores between 0 and 7) represented low levels of photosensitivity-related avoidance behavior. Scores between 8 and 13 represented moderate photosensitivity-related avoidance behavior, and scores equal to or greater than 14 indicated high photosensitivity-related avoidance behavior. As illustrated in Table 2 displaying one-way ANOVA results, the three clinical reference groups (i.e., low, moderate, and high) significantly differed across all measures of construct and criterion validity (e.g., FOPQ-C Total, FOPQ-C Fear subscale, and FOPQ-C Avoidance subscale; HIT-6 Total; SCREEN-SA subscale, PedMIDAS Home and Activities items). Upon examining pair-wise comparisons, for the FOPQ-C total and subscale scores, all tertile groups were significantly different. For the HIT-6, the low group was significantly different from the moderate and high group (but the latter two did not differ). For the SCREEN-SA scale and the PedMIDAS-Home and PedMIDAS-Activities items, only the low and high groups were distinct from each other.

When repeating analyses using quartiles to define the groups, all ANOVAs remained significant; however, examination of pair-wise comparisons yielded far less sensitivity to between-group differences in the selected measures of construct and criterion validity. In particular, the none/minimal and mild groups did not significantly differ from one another across any of the measures examined. Thus, tertile-derived groups were chosen as the more appropriate and parsimonious clinical reference points.

Table 2. One-way ANOVAs between PHOTO-SABS clinical reference groups and validity measures.

	Photosensitivity Avoidance Behavior Reference Group				
	Low	**Moderate**	**High**	*F*	η^2
FOPQ-C Total score	30.48 ^{b,c}	41.84 ^{a,c}	51.75 ^{a,b}	32.80 *	0.28
FOPQ-C Fear subscale score	15.67 ^{b,c}	21.62 ^{a,c}	26.57 ^{a,b}	21.80 *	0.20
FOPQ-C Avoidance subscale score	14.81 ^{b,c}	20.22 ^{a,c}	25.17 ^{a,b}	26.38 *	0.23
HIT-6 Total score	60.86 ^{b,c}	64.55 ^{a}	67.22 ^{a}	18.47 *	0.18
SCREEN School Avoidance	8.14 ^{c}	10.25	11.73 ^{a}	9.39 *	0.10
PedMIDAS—Home Item	11.66 ^{c}	19.28	30.43 ^{a}	9.81 *	0.10
PedMIDAS—Activities Item	13.74 ^{c}	16.38	28.46 ^{a}	5.87 *	0.06

* $p < 0.007$. Within each row, group means with superscripts differ significantly from the other group(s) at $p < 0.007$, after applying a Bonferroni correction (e.g., a (low) is significantly different from b (moderate) and c (high), and so forth). For PHOTO-SABS, sample size for each group was n = 58 (low), n = 55 (moderate), and n = 63 (high).

Regarding demographic factors, there were no significant differences in participant age, sex assigned at birth, gender identity, or race across clinical reference groups, as measured by one-way ANOVAs and chi-square analyses. In terms of pain-related variables, there were no significant differences in photosensitivity-related avoidance behavior based upon headache diagnosis, time since headache onset, headache frequency, and duration of each headache episode. There were significant differences in headache pain intensity ($F = 7.456$, $df = 2$, $p < 0.01$). Inspection of pair-wise comparisons revealed that, while the high- and moderate-avoidance-behavior groups rated their pain intensity significantly higher than the low-avoidance-behavior group, the high- and moderate-avoidance-behavior groups were not significantly different from one another in terms of pain intensity.

3.4. Clinical Reference Points: PHONO-SABS

PHONO-SABS scores in the lowest tertile (i.e., scores between 0 and 5) represented low levels of photosensitivity-related avoidance behavior. Scores between 6 and 13 represented moderate photosensitivity-related avoidance behavior, and scores equal to or higher than 14 represented high photosensitivity-related avoidance behavior. As can be seen in Table 3 displaying one-way ANOVA results, the three clinical reference groups (i.e., low, moderate, and high) significantly differed across all measures of construct and criterion validity (e.g., FOPQ-C Total, FOPQ-C Fear subscale, and FOPQ-C Avoidance subscale; HIT-6 Total; SCREEN-SA subscale, PedMIDAS Home and Activities items). Upon examining pair-wise comparisons, for the FOPQ-C total and subscale scores, all tertile groups were significantly different. For the HIT-6, the low group was significantly different from the moderate and high group (but the latter two did not differ). For the SCREEN-SA scale and the PedMIDAS-Home and PedMIDAS-Activities items, only the low and high groups were distinct from one another.

When repeating analyses using quartiles to define the groups, all ANOVAs remained significant. However, as with the PHOTO-SABS, inspection of pair-wise comparisons in PHONO-SABS quartile groups yielded far less sensitivity to between-group differences in the selected measures of construct and criterion validity. Neither the none/minimal and mild groups nor the moderate and severe groups were significantly different from one another across the majority of the measures examined. Thus, tertile-derived groups were chosen as the more appropriate and parsimonious clinical reference points.

Table 3. One-way ANOVAs between PHONO-SABS clinical reference groups and validity measures.

	Phonosensitivity Avoidance Behavior Reference Group				
	Low	**Moderate**	**High**	*F*	η^2
FOPQ-C Total score	31.24 ^{b,c}	40.85 ^{a,c}	52.66 ^{a,b,c}	32.20 *	0.27
FOPQ-C Fear subscale score	16.22 ^{b,c}	21.22 ^{a,c}	26.76 ^{a,b}	19.29 *	0.18
FOPQ-C Avoidance subscale score	15.02 ^{b,c}	19.63 ^{a,c}	25.90 ^{a,b}	29.09 *	0.25
HIT-6 Total score	61.17 ^{b,c}	64.54 ^{a}	67.10 ^{a}	15.07 *	0.15
SCREEN School Avoidance	8.91 ^{c}	9.63	11.71 ^{a}	5.75 *	0.06
PedMIDAS—Home Item	12.28 ^{c}	20.83	29.12 ^{a}	7.34 *	0.08
PedMIDAS—Activities Item	14.49 ^{c}	16.26	28.69 ^{a}	5.51 *	0.06

* $p < 0.007$. Within each row, group means with superscripts differ significantly from the other group(s) at $p < 0.007$, after applying a Bonferroni correction (e.g., a (low) is significantly different from b (moderate) and c (high), and so forth). For PHONO-SABS, sample size for each group was n = 58 (low), n = 59 (moderate), and n = 59 (high).

Regarding demographic factors, there were no significant differences in participant age, sex assigned at birth, gender identity, or race across clinical reference groups, as measured by one-way ANOVAs and chi-square analyses. In terms of pain-related variables, there were no significant differences in headache diagnosis, time since headache onset, headache frequency, and duration of each headache episode. There were significant differences in headache pain intensity ($F = 6.818$, $df = 2$, $p < 0.01$). Inspection of pairwise comparisons revealed that, while the high- and moderate-avoidance-behavior groups rated their pain intensity significantly higher than the low-avoidance-behavior group, the high- and moderate-avoidance-behavior groups did not significantly differ from one another in reported pain intensity.

3.5. Reliable Change Criterion (RCCrit)

Based upon the standard deviation (7.72) and the reliability estimate (0.91) of the PHOTO-SABS total score, the RCCrit is as follows: $(7.72 \times \sqrt{2} \times \sqrt{1-0.91}) \times 1.96 = 6.4$. Thus, changes in PHOTO-SABS total scores of more than 6.4 can be regarded as reliable changes (e.g., reductions if examining pre- to post-treatment intervention studies) in photosensitivity-related avoidance behavior. Similarly, based upon the standard deviation (8.78) and the reliability estimate (0.93) of the PHONO-SABS total score, the RCCrit is as follows: $(8.78 \times \sqrt{2} \times \sqrt{1-0.93}) \times 1.96 = 6.4$. Thus, changes in PHONO-SABS scores of more than 6.4 can be regarded as reliable changes (e.g., reductions if examining pre- to post-treatment intervention studies) in phonosensitivity-related avoidance behavior.

4. Discussion

This study represents the final phase in the validation of the PhotoSensitivity and PhonoSensitivity Avoidance Behavior Scales (PHOTO-SABS and PHONO-SABS). In the current phase, the authors sought to solidify the prior development [19] and validation [20] of these measures by confirming the scales' psychometric properties, including internal consistency and factor structure. Furthermore, the authors also sought to expand the measures' clinical utility by establishing clinical reference points and determining the reliable change criterion for each measure. These findings will allow clinicians to more clearly interpret the meaning of various scores on these measures as well as to assess clinically meaningful changes after intervention in youth who experience visual and auditory sensitivities with their primary chronic headaches.

4.1. Review of Findings

The 11-item PHOTO-SABS retained its same two-factor structure as the original measure validation study [20], with subscales measuring Changes to Participation and

Modification of Environment. The total score and subscale scores of the PHOTO-SABS demonstrated strong internal consistency and strong factor loadings therein. Similarly, the 12-item PHONO-SABS retained its same structure, a single factor with no subscales. The total score of the PHONO-SABS exhibited excellent internal consistency and strong factor loadings.

The importance of having dedicated, specialized psychometrically sound assessment tools to guide research endeavors, particularly in pediatric headache, cannot be understated. These findings confirm, in a novel sample, what previous work has demonstrated: the PHOTO-SABS and PHONO-SABS are feasible, acceptable, sound, valid measures of previously understudied phenomena in pediatric chronic headaches. As noted previously, prior to the development of the PHOTO-SABS and PHONO-SABS, not only were there no validated measures of sensory sensitivity-related avoidance behavior, but there was also little investigation into photo- and phonosensitivity in pediatric headache and related behavior, beyond the presence/absence of the symptom. As researchers and clinicians learn more about the role of central sensitization [10] across pediatric chronic pain conditions, it appears crucial to understand the associated symptoms that may also contribute to functional disability. Further, while there are measures of pediatric pain-related fear and avoidance (e.g., FOPQ-C [16]), the PHOTO-SABS and PHONO-SABS explore beyond avoidance of movement and of pain to capture nuanced aspects of the pediatric chronic headache experience.

The key indices of clinical utility established here, clinical reference groups and an RC-Crit for each measure, can further aid in the interpretation and application of PHOTO-SABS and PHONO-SABS scores. The clinical reference groups (tertiles labeled low, moderate, and high) were robustly sensitive in detecting differences across all measures of construct and criterion validity, with medium to very large effects across all variables of interest (η^2 = 0.06–0.28 for the PHOTO-SABS and 0.06–0.27 for the PHONO-SABS). At the pair-wise level, this demonstrated the need for global measures of avoidance and functional impact but was less apparent for domain-specific items. Here, there were fewer significant differences between the low/moderate and moderate/high groups, suggesting that at the level of specific domains (e.g., school, home, social life/activities) in avoidance behavior scores may present more dichotomously. This is consistent with the smaller effects here vs. larger effects with measures more directly assessing avoidance behavior and global impact. Ultimately, these findings suggest that the clinical reference groups are applicable in research settings in cross-sectional research studies to classify patients as having low, moderate, or high levels of sensitivity-related avoidance behavior. They can also be used in clinical assessment to not only enhance understanding of the headache experience, but also to match patients with appropriate interventions and stratify patients into the suitable level of care. For instance, patients with high scores on the PHOTO- and PHONO-SABs may necessitate targeted desensitization interventions such as those offered in more intensive pain rehabilitation programs. On the other hand, those with low scores may benefit from education alone, perhaps on the Fear-Avoidance Model (FAM) of Chronic Pain [14]. Moreover, the RCCrit calculated for each of the two measures can be used to assess clinically meaningful change, an area often overlooked in the developmental of new measurement tools, particularly in pediatric chronic pain [33]. However, the potential applications of the RCCrit are innumerable, as it allows researchers and clinicians to determine whether the changes observed in treatment outcome studies and in day-to-day practice are clinically meaningful.

4.2. Implications for Clinical Practice

The PHOTO-SABS and PHONO-SABS are practical measures that can be administered in under three minutes, making them highly feasible for routine clinical use and in research settings [19]. Their ease of administration and interpretation allows for utilization by a wide range of health care professionals, across disciplines and with varying degrees of specificity in their practice. For instance, data gleaned from the PHOTO-SABS and PHONO-SABS have clinical relevance for care provided by headache specialists, such as pain physicians, neurologists, psychologists, and allied health practitioners (e.g., occupational and physical therapists). Clinicians are encouraged to incorporate the PHOTO-SABS and PHONO-SABS into their initial evaluations to assess avoidance related to sensory sensitivities, which may otherwise not be identified through closed-ended, dichotomous questions, such as, "Do you have sensitivity to lights or sounds?" At the same time, the PHOTO-SABS and PHONO-SAB can also be used by primary care physicians, who are often the first-line providers helping patients to assess persistent headaches. These measures can be implemented as brief screening tools to help pediatricians detect patients who may benefit from further neurological evaluation and/or specialized headache-related care. In fact, such tools may provide pediatricians with the data needed to justify a multidisciplinary approach to care for chronic headaches.

The PHOTO-SABS and the PHONO-SABS also complement the existing assessment tools typically included in headache clinic batteries, such as the HIT-6 [25,26], PedMIDAS [28], and FOPQ-C [16]. The addition of measures assessing the impact of sensory sensitivities on functioning facilitates a more comprehensive evaluation of the headache experience. By revealing nuanced and typically subtle avoidance behaviors, the PHOTO-SABS and PHONO-SABS provide valuable insights that can enhance treatment planning across disciplines and inform the selection of targeted interventions, ensuring a client-centered and individualized approach to care.

4.3. Limitations

This study is not without limitations, which warrant careful consideration. While the sample demographics in this study generally align with youth patients presenting to this tertiary multidisciplinary headache clinic in the Northeast, the sample was notably homogenous. Future research should aim to diversify sample characteristics, specifically focusing on sex assigned at birth, gender identity, race, and ethnicity, to enhance the generalizability of these findings and ensure that they reflect the experience of all youth with primary chronic headaches. Moreover, due to the self-reported nature of the PHOTO-SABS and PHONO-SABS, responses are inherently subject to potential response bias and the limited introspective capacity of respondents, particularly younger participants. To mitigate these risks, it is advisable to pair self-reported measures with clinical observations from clinicians and/or caregiver input. Future studies might also explore the development of separate caregiver proxy measures to complement youth self-reports. Additionally, it is important to acknowledge that data were collected electronically prior to the clinic visit, requiring respondents to engage in cognitive activity and interact with a screen. Particularly for individuals with photosensitivity, caregiver assistance to complete the measures may have introduced bias or influence upon youth responses. Further investigation of this measure could consider utilizing multiple methods of data collection (e.g., electronic, pencil/paper, or verbal) and/or data collection within the clinic setting to minimize this limitation and better accommodate diverse respondent needs.

4.4. Future Directions

The conceptualization of this measure development study emerged from an identified gap in the literature: no existing measures had been available to assess avoidance behavior in youth with primary chronic headaches who experience photo- and phonosensitivity. Following the development and initial validation of the PHOTO-SABS and PHONO-SABS, these tools have already been successfully integrated into multidisciplinary headache care and intensive interdisciplinary pain rehabilitation settings. With the measures' clinical utility substantiated in this study, researchers now have valuable, methodologically sound resources to formally assess clinical changes in avoidance behaviors related to photo- and phonosensitivity. Continued application will help to disseminate their utility across settings and disciplines, particularly in the initial assessment and in setting treatment goals for functional rehabilitation. Now, with clinical reference points and the reliable change criterion, a novel application for these measures is the assessment of meaningful change in sensitivity-related avoidance behavior during and after participation in interventions focused on desensitization.

There are myriad potential extensions of the current measures, which could include exploring differences in sensitivity-related avoidance behavior across pediatric headache presentations. While photo- and phonosensitivity are typically most associated with pediatric migraine [36], anecdotally in the clinic and as evidenced in our three measure validation studies, it appears that such sensitivities are reported to be very much present in all primary chronic headaches experienced by youth. Understanding any nuances in those experiences could help to further individualize treatment approaches and identify potential barriers to functioning. Relatedly, another extension of these findings could be to explore sensory sensitivity-related avoidance behavior in non-headache pain conditions. Given the role of central sensitization of the nervous system in all manifestations of chronic pain [37], it is possible and even likely that youth with other types of persistent pain conditions could also experience sensory sensitivity-related avoidance behavior that contributes to their functional disability.

Replication of these validation studies and additional examination of their use in more diverse samples (with regard to demographics and headache characteristics) is a future direction to consider, as noted earlier. Further, given that primary chronic headaches can present and persist across the lifespan, future research could adapt and validate these measures in young adults and adults. Modifications to the current tools is warranted, such as replacing school-related items with those that pertain to job or work environments, to ensure broader applicability in these age groups. This would not only extend the utility of the measures but also enhance their relevance in diverse settings beyond the pediatric population.

4.5. Conclusions

The PHOTO- and PHONO-SABS are theoretically driven, psychometrically validated, clinically useful measures for assessing sensory sensitivity-related avoidance behavior in youth with primary chronic headaches. These measures offer unique insights by capturing how photo- and phonosensitivity, beyond pain, can contribute qualitatively to avoidance behavior, ultimately impacting developmentally appropriate functioning across multiple domains. By establishing clinical reference points, clinicians can better interpret scores on these measures, further quantify the degree of sensitivity-related avoidance behavior, and understand its deleterious impact on participation in daily activities. Furthermore, in determining the reliable change criteria, clinicians can monitor changes in avoidance behavior over time, perhaps to understand parallel changes in functioning or to assess responses to various interventions (e.g., auditory and visual desensitization). The PHOTO-SABS and PHOTO-SABS now allow clinicians to measure and track meaningful changes in sensitivity-related avoidance behavior in both clinical and research settings to improve outcomes for youth with primary chronic headaches.

Author Contributions: Conceptualization, M.N.S.; methodology, A.M.S.; software, A.M.S.; formal analysis, A.M.S.; investigation, A.M.S. and M.N.S.; data curation, H.R.; writing—original draft preparation, A.M.S. and M.N.S.; writing—review and editing, H.R. and A.A.L.; supervision, A.M.S. and A.A.L. All authors have read and agreed to the published version of the manuscript.

Funding: This research received no external funding.

Institutional Review Board Statement: The study was conducted in accordance with the Declaration of Helsinki and approved by the Institutional Review Board of Boston Children's Hospital (IRB-IRB-P00030246).

Informed Consent Statement: Patient consent was waived as the data were initially collected as part of clinical practice and stored in a clinical data repository. Therefore, all retrospective studies using data from the data repository have approval for waiver of consent by our IRB.

Data Availability Statement: The data presented in this study are available on request from the corresponding author. The data are not publicly available due to the privacy policies in place at the institution at which the data were collected.

Acknowledgments: The authors would like to acknowledge the Boston Children's Hospital Chronic Pain Data Repository team, which manages the clinical data collected within the Division of Pain Medicine in the Department of Anesthesiology, including all data used in this study, especially Carolina Donado, for her support with dataset construction, management, and analytics. The authors would also like to acknowledge Christopher Butler, the developer and manager of the web-based platform for data collection that has become part of our clinical standard of care.

Conflicts of Interest: The authors declare no conflicts of interest.

References

1. Chambers, C.T.; Dol, J.; Tutelman, P.R.; Langley, C.L.; Parker, J.A.; Cormier, B.T.; Macfarlane, G.J.; Jones, G.T.; Chapman, D.; Proudfoot, N.; et al. The prevalence of chronic pain in children and adolescents: A systematic review update and meta-analysis. *Pain* **2024**, *165*, 2215–2234. [CrossRef]
2. Pawlowski, C.; Buckman, C.; Tumin, D.; Smith, A.W.; Crotty, J. National trends in pediatric headache and associated functional limitations. *Clin. Pediatr.* **2019**, *58*, 1502–1508. [CrossRef]
3. Hershey, A.D. What is the impact, prevalence, disability, and quality of life of pediatric headache? *Curr. Pain Headache Rep.* **2005**, *9*, 341–344. [CrossRef]
4. Shulman, J.; Conroy, C.; Cybulski, A.; Smith, K.R.; Jervis, K.; Johnson, H.; Zurakowski, D.; Sethna, N.F. Does intensive interdisciplinary pain treatment improve pediatric headache-related disability? *Disabil. Rehabilitation* **2020**, *44*, 194–201. [CrossRef]
5. Bellini, B.; Arruda, M.; Cescut, A.; Saulle, C.; Persico, A.; Carotenuto, M.; Gatta, M.; Nacinovich, R.; Piazza, F.P.; Termine, C.; et al. Headache and comorbidity in children and adolescents. *J. Headache Pain* **2013**, *14*, 79. [CrossRef]
6. Law, E.F.; Palermo, T.M.; Zhou, C.; Groenewald, C.B. Economic impact of headache and psychiatric comorbidities on healthcare expenditures among children in the United States: A retrospective cross-sectional study. *Headache J. Head Face Pain* **2019**, *59*, 1504–1515. [CrossRef]
7. Powers, S.W.; Patton, S.R.; Hommel, K.A.; Hershey, A.D. Quality of life in childhood migraines: Clinical impact and comparison to other chronic illnesses. *Pediatrics* **2003**, *112*, e1–e5. [CrossRef]
8. Reidy, B.L.; Riddle, E.J.; Powers, S.W.; Slater, S.K.; Kacperski, J.; Kabbouche, M.A.; Hershey, A.D. Clinic-based characterization of continuous headache in children and adolescents: Comparing youth with chronic migraine to those with new daily persistent headache. *Cephalalgia* **2020**, *40*, 1063–1069. [CrossRef]
9. Genizi, J.; Halevy, A.; Schertz, M.; Osman, K.; Assaf, N.; Segal, I.; Srugo, I.; Kessel, A.; Engel-Yeger, B. Altered sensory processing patterns correlate with disease severity and quality of life among children with migraine. *Front. Neurol.* **2019**, *10*, 448. [CrossRef]
10. de Tommaso, M.; Sciruicchio, V.; Delussi, M.; Vecchio, E.; Goffredo, M.; Simeone, M.; Barbaro, M.G.F. Symptoms of central sensitization and comorbidity for juvenile fibromyalgia in childhood migraine: An observational study in a tertiary headache center. *J. Headache Pain* **2017**, *18*, 1–10. [CrossRef]
11. Nahman-Averbuch, H.; Leon, E.; Hunter, B.M.; Ding, L.; Hershey, A.D.; Powers, S.W.; King, C.D.; Coghill, R.C. Increased pain sensitivity but normal pain modulation in adolescents with migraine. *Pain* **2019**, *160*, 1019–1028. [CrossRef]
12. Neut, D.; Fily, A.; Cuvellier, J.-C.; Vallée, L. The prevalence of triggers in paediatric migraine: A questionnaire study in 102 children and adolescents. *J. Headache Pain* **2011**, *13*, 61–65. [CrossRef]
13. Strong, E.; Pierce, E.L.; Langdon, R.; Strelzik, J.; McClintock, W.; Cameron, M.; Furda, M.; DiSabella, M. New Daily Persistent Headache in a Pediatric Population. *J. Child Neurol.* **2021**, *36*, 888–893. [CrossRef]
14. Vlaeyen, J.W.S.; Linton, S.J. Fear-avoidance and its consequences in chronic musculoskeletal pain: A state of the art. *Pain* **2000**, *85*, 317–332. [CrossRef]
15. Simons, L.E.; Kaczynski, K.J. The fear avoidance model of chronic pain: Examination for pediatric application. *J. Pain* **2012**, *13*, 827–835. [CrossRef]
16. Simons, L.E.; Sieberg, C.B.; Carpino, E.; Logan, D.; Berde, C. The Fear of Pain Questionnaire (FOPQ): Assessment of pain-related fear among children and adolescents with chronic pain. *J. Pain* **2011**, *12*, 677–686. [CrossRef]
17. E Simons, L.; Pielech, M.; Cappucci, S.; Lebel, A. Fear of pain in pediatric headache. *Cephalalgia* **2014**, *35*, 36–44. [CrossRef]
18. Glogan, E.; Meulders, M.; Pfeiffer, L.; Vlaeyen, J.W.; Meulders, A. Alike, But Not Quite: Comparing the Generalization of Pain-Related Fear and Pain-Related Avoidance. *J. Pain* **2022**, *23*, 1616–1628. [CrossRef]
19. Silvia, M.; Smith, A.M. Development and Feasibility of the Headache-Related Light and Sound Sensitivity Inventories in Youth. *Children* **2021**, *8*, 861. [CrossRef]
20. Smith, A.M.; Silvia, M.; Rogan, H.; Schefter, Z.J. Avoiding lights and sounds: Validation of the PhotoSensitivity and PhonoSensitivity Avoidance Behavior Scales (PHOTO-SABS & PHONO-SABS) in pediatric headache. *Child. Health Care* **2023**, *53*, 76–95. [CrossRef]
21. Headache Classification Committee of the International Headache Society (IHS) The International Classification of Headache Disorders, 3rd edition. *Cephalalgia Int. J. Headache* **2018**, *38*, 1–211. [CrossRef]

22. Silberstein, S.D.; Dodick, D.W.; Pearlman, S. Defining the pharmacologically intractable headache for clinical trials and clinical practice. *Headache J. Head Face Pain* **2010**, *50*, 1499–1506. [CrossRef]
23. Seshia, S.S. Mixed migraine and tension-type: A common cause of recurrent headache in children. *Can. J. Neurol. Sci. J. Can. Sci. Neurol.* **2004**, *31*, 315–318. [CrossRef]
24. von Baeyer, C.L.; Spagrud, L.J.; McCormick, J.C.; Choo, E.; Neville, K.; Connelly, M.A. Three new datasets supporting use of the Numerical Rating Scale (NRS-11) for children's self-reports of pain intensity. *Pain* **2009**, *143*, 223–227. [CrossRef]
25. Kosinski, M.; Bayliss, M.S.; Bjorner, J.B.; Ware, J.E.; Garber, W.; Batenhorst, A.; Cady, R.; Dahlöf, C.; Dowson, A.; Tepper, S. A six-item short-form survey for measuring headache impact: The HIT-6™. *Qual. Life Res.* **2003**, *12*, 963–974. [CrossRef]
26. Piebes, S.K.; Snyder, A.R.; Bay, R.C.; McLeod, T.C.V. Measurement properties of headache-specific outcomes scales in adolescent athletes. *J. Sport Rehabilitation* **2011**, *20*, 129–142. [CrossRef]
27. Gallé-Tessonneau, M.; Gana, K. Development and Validation of the School Refusal Evaluation Scale1 for Adolescents. *J. Pediatr. Psychol.* **2018**, *44*, 153–163. [CrossRef]
28. Hershey, A.D.; Powers, S.W.; Vockell, A.-L.B.; LeCates, S.; Kabbouche, M.; Maynard, M.K. PedMIDAS: Development of a questionnaire to assess disability of migraines in children. *Neurology* **2001**, *57*, 2034–2039. [CrossRef]
29. Donado, C.; Lobo, K.; Berde, C.B.; Bourgeois, F.T. Developing a pediatric pain data repository. *JAMIA Open* **2020**, *3*, 31–36. [CrossRef]
30. Hu, L.T.; Bentler, P.M. Cutoff criteria for fit indexes in covariance structure analysis: Conventional criteria versus new alternatives. *Struct. Equ. Model. Multidiscip. J.* **1999**, *6*, 1–55. [CrossRef]
31. Kline, R.B. *Principles and Practice of Structural Equation Modeling*, 2nd ed.; Guilford: New York, NY, USA, 2005.
32. Pielech, M.; Ryan, M.; Logan, D.; Kaczynski, K.; White, M.T.; Simons, L.E. Pain catastrophizing in children with chronic pain and their parents: Proposed clinical reference points and reexamination of the Pain Catastrophizing Scale measure. *Pain* **2014**, *155*, 2360–2367. [CrossRef]
33. Heathcote, L.C.; Bhandari, R.P.; Timmers, I.; Harrison, L.E.; Simons, L.E. Rapid identification and clinical indices of fear-avoidance in youth with chronic pain. *Pain* **2019**, *161*, 565–573. [CrossRef]
34. Stone, A.L.; Walker, L.S.; Heathcote, L.C.; Hernandez, J.M.; Basch, M.C.; Wilson, A.C.; Simons, L.E. Somatic symptoms in pediatric patients with chronic pain: Proposed clinical reference points for the children's somatic symptoms inventory (formerly the children's somatization inventory). *J. Pain* **2019**, *20*, 932–940. [CrossRef]
35. Sil, S.; Arnold, L.M.; Lynch-Jordan, A.; Ting, T.V.; Peugh, J.; Cunningham, N.; Powers, S.W.; Lovell, D.J.; Hashkes, P.J.; Passo, M.; et al. Identifying treatment responders and predictors of improvement after cognitive-behavioral therapy for juvenile fibromyalgia. *Pain* **2014**, *155*, 1206–1212. [CrossRef]
36. Kim, S. Pediatric headache: A narrative review. *J. Yeungnam Med. Sci.* **2022**, *39*, 278–284. [CrossRef]
37. Nijs, J.; George, S.Z.; Clauw, D.J.; Fernández-De-Las-Peñas, C.; Kosek, E.; Ickmans, K.; Fernández-Carnero, J.; Polli, A.; Kapreli, E.; Huysmans, E.; et al. Central sensitisation in chronic pain conditions: Latest discoveries and their potential for precision medicine. *Lancet Rheumatol.* **2021**, *3*, e383–e392. [CrossRef]

children

MDPI

Article

Clinical and Multivariate Predictors of Headaches Attributed to Rhinosinusitis in Pediatric Patients: A Comparative Study with Migraine and Tension-Type Headache

Seung Beom Han [1,2], Eu Gene Park [1,3] and Ji Yoon Han [1,4,*]

1 Department of Pediatrics, College of Medicine, The Catholic University of Korea, Seoul 06591, Republic of Korea; beomsid@catholic.ac.kr (S.B.H.); eugene.park@catholic.ac.kr (E.G.P.)
2 Department of Pediatrics, Bucheon St. Mary's Hospital, College of Medicine, The Catholic University of Korea, Bucheon 14647, Republic of Korea
3 Department of Pediatrics, Incheon St. Mary's Hospital, College of Medicine, The Catholic University of Korea, Incheon 21431, Republic of Korea
4 Department of Pediatrics, Daejeon St. Mary's Hospital, College of Medicine, The Catholic University of Korea, Daejeon 34943, Republic of Korea
* Correspondence: han024@catholic.ac.kr; Tel.: +82-42-220-9540

Highlights

What are the main findings?

- Pediatric headache attributed to rhinosinusitis (HRS) was often misdiagnosed as migraine or tension-type headache, especially in younger children.
- Multivariate analysis identified distinct predictors of HRS, including nasal and auditory symptoms, allergic rhinitis, and family history of HRS.

What are the implications of the main finding?

- Incorporating otolaryngologic and allergic features into diagnostic evaluation can improve accuracy and reduce misclassification.
- These predictors may help clinicians avoid unnecessary neuroimaging and provide timely, targeted therapy for pediatric patients.

Abstract

Background/Objectives: Headache attributed to rhinosinusitis (HRS) is uncommon in children but often misdiagnosed as migraine or tension-type headache (TTH). Overlapping phenotypes, incidental sinus findings on neuroimaging, and limited communication in younger patients complicate diagnosis and lead to inappropriate treatment. Methods: We retrospectively analyzed 3065 pediatric patients (<19 years) presenting with headache at two tertiary neurology clinics (2014–2023) with $\geq$1 year follow-up. Headaches were classified by ICHD-3 criteria. HRS diagnosis required radiologic sinus pathology and $\geq$50% improvement within 72 h of antibiotic or decongestant therapy. Demographic, clinical, neuroimaging, and family history data were collected. Symptom profiling used principal component analysis (PCA) and k-means clustering; multivariate logistic regression identified independent predictors. Results: Of 3065 patients, 32.7% had migraines, 15.5% TTH, and 4.5% HRS. Nearly one-third of HRS cases were initially misclassified. Compared with migraine and TTH, HRS patients were younger (median 9 years), more often male, and enriched in preschool age. Independent predictors included shorter duration (<1 h; OR 0.62), higher intensity (OR 2.165), nasal symptoms (OR 9.836), hearing impairment (OR 22.52), allergic rhinitis (OR 8.468), and family history of HRS (OR 32.602) (all $p < 0.001$). PCA showed overlap but distinct clustering: HRS was characterized by sinonasal and otologic features, whereas migraine clustered around sensory hypersensitivity. Conclusions: Pediatric HRS shows distinct predictors—young age, acute severe headache, nasal and auditory symptoms, allergic history, and family history—despite overlap with migraine and TTH. Structured use of these predictors with otolaryngologic assessment may improve diagnostic accuracy, reduce misclassification, and avoid unnecessary neuroimaging or inappropriate therapy.

Keywords: headache attributed to rhinosinusitis; migraine; tension-type headache

1. Introduction

Headache attributed to rhinosinusitis (HRS) is relatively uncommon in pediatric and adolescent populations, with an estimated diagnostic rate ranging from 3% to 11% among headache sufferers [1–4]. In comparison, primary headache disorders such as migraine and tension-type headache (TTH) are considerably more prevalent. Meta-analytic data indicate that migraine affects approximately 11% of children and adolescents, while TTH has a pooled prevalence of around 17% [5–8]. Although the International Classification of Headache Disorders (ICHD-3) provides distinct diagnostic criteria, clinical differentiation of headache subtypes in children often remains challenging due to overlapping symptoms, age-dependent expression of pain, and limited communication ability [9].

Misdiagnosis is particularly common between HRS and primary headache disorders, with studies reporting that up to 50–80% of pediatric patients initially diagnosed with sinus-related headaches were later reclassified as having migraine or TTH after specialist evaluation [10,11]. Furthermore, incidental paranasal sinus abnormalities on neuroimaging are detected in up to 30% of asymptomatic children, contributing to diagnostic uncertainty and frequent inappropriate antibiotic use [12,13].

Migraine in pediatric patients may present with bilateral pain, short duration, and more prominent gastrointestinal symptoms compared to adults, whereas TTH typically manifests with pressure-like pain and fewer autonomic features [2,14]. HRS are frequently associated with facial pain or pressure, nasal symptoms, and positional aggravation, but its phenotypic overlap with migraine and TTH often obscures accurate diagnosis in routine practice. Given these diagnostic ambiguities, reliance solely on conventional clinical criteria may lead to misclassification and suboptimal treatment. Recent studies have advocated for a data-driven approach to headache classification, incorporating symptom profiling, cluster analysis, and machine learning techniques to better define phenotypic subgroups beyond traditional diagnostic boundaries [13,15]. The distinction between headache attributed to rhinosinusitis (HRS) and primary headaches such as migraine and tension-type headache was clarified based on the ICHD-3 criteria. HRS typically presents with dull or pressure-like pain associated with nasal symptoms, whereas migraine is characterized by pulsating pain with sensory hypersensitivity.

Therefore, this study aimed to comprehensively analyze the clinical characteristics of pediatric patients with migraine, TTH, and HRS. In addition, we sought to identify multivariate clinical and symptom-based predictors that can effectively distinguish HRS from primary headache disorders, thereby improving diagnostic precision and facilitating appropriate clinical management

2. Materials and Methods

2.1. Study Design and Participants

This retrospective cohort study included pediatric patients who visited the pediatric neurology outpatient clinics of Incheon St. Mary's Hospital and Daejeon St. Mary's

Hospital, affiliated with the Catholic University of Korea, from March 2014 to December 2023. To ensure diagnostic accuracy and clinical relevance, only patients with at least 1 year of follow-up after their initial visit were included. Data extraction and verification were performed independently by two pediatric neurologists using a standardized case report form. Any discrepancies in classification or variable coding were resolved by consensus review to minimize diagnostic bias and ensure reproducibility. Eligible participants were children and adolescents (<19 years) presenting with headache as their primary complaint and undergoing standardized headache assessment including detailed clinical history, neurological examination, and neuroimaging.

Exclusion criteria were (1) known systemic diseases (e.g., autoimmune, metabolic, or oncologic disorders), (2) intracranial space-occupying lesions, (3) significant head trauma within 3 months prior to the initial visit, (4) neurologic disorders unrelated to primary headache, (5) chronic use of medications known to affect headache characteristics (e.g., corticosteroids, valproic acid, or tricyclic antidepressants), (6) secondary headache disorders other than rhinosinusitis, (7) incomplete medical records or <1 year of follow-up, and (8) developmental or cognitive disorders precluding reliable symptom reporting.

2.2. Data Collection and Variables

Demographic and clinical data were extracted from electronic medical records, including age, sex, headache onset pattern, duration, pain location, and intensity (assessed using a 0–10 numeric rating scale), frequency, associated symptoms (e.g., gastrointestinal symptoms such as nausea/vomiting; neurological manifestations including visual disturbances and dizziness), headache triggers (e.g., sleep deprivation or specific foods), allergy history (e.g., allergic rhinitis, or asthma), and family history of migraine or other headache disorders. Neuroimaging findings (brain MRI or CT) were reviewed where available. Sinusitis was radiologically confirmed by mucosal thickening $\geq$ 3 mm or air-fluid levels in the paranasal sinuses, and findings were graded using the Lund-Mackay scoring system when applicable. Cases with missing key data (<5%) were excluded from variable-specific analyses. Headache duration was defined as the typical attack length reported by the patient or caregiver. Pain intensity was measured on a 0–10 scale and classified as mild (1–3), moderate (4–6), or severe (7–10). Other categorical variables such as pain type and triggers were coded as present (1) or absent (0) for analysis.

2.3. Headache Classification

Headaches were classified according to ICHD-3. A diagnosis HRS required (1) a temporal relationship between headache onset and documented sinus pathology, defined as radiologic evidence of mucosal thickening $\geq$ 3 mm or air-fluid levels on paranasal sinus imaging, and (2) $\geq$50% reduction in headache severity within 72 h of antibiotic or decongestant therapy. Cases without adequate clinical–radiologic correlation or therapeutic response were categorized into the non-HRS group, comprising migraine and TTH based on ICHD-3 criteria. All classifications were independently reviewed by two pediatric neurologists, with discrepancies resolved by consensus.

2.4. Statistical and Analytical Methods

Symptom profiles were binarized (present = 1, absent = 0), with missing values (<5%) imputed as absent. Normality of continuous variables was assessed using the Shapiro–Wilk test, and appropriate parametric (Student's *t*-test) or non-parametric (Mann–Whitney U) tests were applied. Continuous variables were summarized as mean $\pm$ SD or median (IQR). Group differences were assessed using appropriate parametric or non-parametric tests

(Student's *t*-test, Mann–Whitney U test, chi-square, or Fisher's exact test) with Bonferroni correction applied to adjust for multiple comparisons. Principal component analysis (PCA) and k-means clustering were applied to identify data-driven headache subtypes independent of diagnostic labels, and the first two principal components were visualized.

Multivariate logistic regression was used to identify independent predictors of HRS, adjusting for clinically relevant covariates (sex, age at diagnosis, headache localization, duration, frequency, intensity, associated symptoms, and family history). Multicollinearity was assessed using VIF (threshold > 5), and model fit was evaluated using the Hosmer–Lemeshow test. Odds ratios (ORs) with 95% confidence intervals (CIs) and *p*-values were reported. Effect sizes were not calculated because most variables were categorical or non-normally distributed. Model fit was checked by the Hosmer–Lemeshow test, and collinearity by VIF (<5). Analyses were conducted using IBM SPSS Statistics v21.0 (IBM Corp., Armonk, NY, USA) and Python v3.11 (Python Software Foundation, Wilmington, DE, USA), with $p < 0.05$ considered statistically significant.

2.5. Ethical Considerations

This study was approved by the Institutional Review Board (IRB) of the Catholic Medical Center (OC23RASI0159 and DC24RASI0047; Seoul, Republic of Korea) and conducted in accordance with the Declaration of Helsinki and ICH-GCP guidelines. The IRB granted a waiver of informed consent due to the retrospective nature of the study and the use of anonymized data to ensure patient confidentiality.

3. Results

3.1. Study Population

A total of 3065 pediatric patients with headache were included (1409 males and 1656 females). The median age at diagnosis was 11 years (interquartile range [IQR]: 8–14; range: 2–19). Among these, 32.7% were diagnosed with migraine, 15.5% with TTH, and 4.5% with HRS. For subgroup analyses, 1140 migraine patients, 474 TTH patients, and 137 HRS patients were compared (Tables 1 and 2). Of the 137 patients ultimately diagnosed with HRS, 13 (27.7%) were initially misclassified as having primary headache disorders, including migraine (n = 10, 21.3%) and TTH (n = 4, 6.4%).

Table 1. Comparison of headache characteristics between the migraine and HRS.

Clinical Characteristics	Migraine (n = 1140)	HRS (n = 137)	*p*-Value
Male (n, %)	471 (41.3)	118 (58.1%)	<0.001
Female (n, %)	669 (58.7)	85 (41.9%)	
Age (years), median (range)	12 (2–18)	9 (3–17)	<0.001
Age at diagnosis (n, %)			<0.001
Pre-school age (≤6 years)	81 (7.1)	39 (28.5)	<0.001
Children (7–12 years)	450 (39.5)	78 (56.9)	<0.001
Adolescent (13–18 years)	609 (53.4)	20 (14.6)	<0.001
Onset type (n, %)			<0.001
Acute (≤3 months)	221 (19.4)	43 (31.4)	0.002
Acute recurrent (≤3 months)	227 (19.9)	19 (13.9)	0.114
Chronic non-progressive (>3 months)	214 (18.8)	50 (36.5)	<0.001

Table 1. *Cont.*

Clinical Characteristics	Migraine (n = 1140)	HRS (n = 137)	*p*-Value
Chronic progressive (>3 months)	478 (41.9)	25 (18.2)	<0.001
Localization (n, %)			<0.001
Diffuse	144 (12.6)	20 (14.6)	0.607
Localized	956 (83.9)	97 (70.8)	<0.001
Mixed	40 (3.5)	20 (14.6)	<0.001
Duration (n, %)			<0.001
<30 min	146 (12.8)	38 (27.7)	<0.001
30–<60 min	141 (12.4)	35 (25.6)	<0.001
≥1 h	853 (74.8)	64 (46.7)	<0.001
Frequency (n, %)			<0.001
<2/month	131 (11.5)	0	<0.001
2–<4/month	248 (21.8)	49 (35.8)	<0.001
4–<15/month	298 (26.2)	50 (36.5)	0.013
≥15/month	161 (14.1)	38 (27.7)	<0.001
Daily	151 (13.2)	0	<0.001
Intensity (n, %)			0.039
Mild	80 (7.0)	18 (13.1)	0.018
Moderate	749 (65.7)	83 (60.6)	0.274
Severe	311 (27.3)	36 (26.3)	0.883
Sleep disturbance due to headache (n, %)	158 (13.9)	22 (16.1)	0.569
Morning headache (n, %)	368 (32.3)	33 (24.1)	0.064
Characteristics (n, %)			<0.001
Throbbing	727 (63.8)	34 (24.8)	<0.001
Sharp	80 (7.0)	9 (6.6)	0.986
Cramping	24 (2.1)	1 (0.7)	0.440
Prickling	105 (9.2)	10 (7.3)	0.562
Constant/dull	33 (2.9)	10 (7.3)	0.014
Pressure	192 (16.8)	33 (24.1)	0.047
Mixed	34 (3.0)	39 (28.5)	<0.001
Others	49 (4.3)	1 (0.7)	0.072
Accompanied symptoms (n, %)	998 (87.5)	78 (56.9)	<0.001
Nausea/vomiting	796 (69.8)	69 (50.4)	<0.001
Abdominal pain	66 (5.8)	15 (11.0)	0.031
Photophobia	266 (23.3)	12 (8.8)	<0.001
Phonophobia	279 (24.5)	0	<0.001
Dizziness	394 (34.6)	44 (32.1)	0.653
Nasal symptoms *	21 (1.8)	53 (38.7)	<0.001
Neurologic manifestations (n, %)	286 (25.1)	30 (21.9)	<0.001
Gait disturbance	1 (0.09)	2 (1.5)	0.028
Focal weakness	33 (2.9)	3 (2.2)	0.843
Visual disturbance	224 (19.6)	26 (19)	0.942
Auditory symptoms #	10 (0.9)	10 (7.3)	<0.001
Dysarthria/aphasia	9 (0.8)	1 (0.7)	1.000
Dysesthesia	38 (3.3)	2 (2.5)	0.352
Decreased consciousness	10 (0.9)	2 (2.5)	0.842
Seizure	3 (0.3)	0	1.000
Movement symptom †	17 (1.5)	4 (2.9)	0.375
Triggering factors (n, %)	266 (23.3)	25 (18.2)	<0.001
Emotional stress	182 (16.0)	15 (11.0)	0.158
Hunger	7 (0.6)	0	0.759
Weather	37 (3.2)	2 (2.5)	0.376
Fatigue	43 (3.8)	15 (11.0)	<0.001

Table 1. *Cont.*

Clinical Characteristics	Migraine (n = 1140)	HRS (n = 137)	*p*-Value
Exercise	17 (1.5)	4 (2.9)	0.375
Light	11 (1.0)	2 (1.5)	0.924
Noise	8 (0.7)	0	0.681
Smell	16 (1.4)	0	0.323
Season at diagnosis (n, %)			0.694
Spring	288 (25.3)	35 (25.6)	1.000
Summer	365 (32.0)	45 (32.8)	0.921
Fall	296 (26.0)	30 (21.9)	0.353
Winter	191 (16.7)	27 (19.7)	0.454
Family history of migraine (n, %)	368 (32.3)	9 (6.6)	<0.001
Family history of TTH (n, %)	45 (3.9)	3 (2.2)	0.008
Family history of HRS (n, %)	12 (1.0)	36 (26.3)	<0.001
Family history of allergic rhinitis (n, %)	23 (2.0)	20 (14.6)	<0.001

† Tremor, myoclonus; * Rhinorrhea, nasal stuffiness, postnasal drip, snoring; # Ear fullness, tinnitus. TTH: tension-type headache, HRS: headache attributed to acute rhinosinusitis. *p*-values were derived using chi-square or Fisher's exact tests for categorical variables and Mann–Whitney U or *t*-tests for continuous variables, as appropriate.

Table 2. Comparison of headache characteristics between the tension-type headache and HRS.

Clinical Characteristics	TTH (n = 474)	HRS (n = 137)	*p*-Value
Male, (n, %)	232 (48.9)	118 (58.1%)	0.035
Female, (n, %)	242 (51.1)	85 (41.9%)	
Age (years), median (range)	11 (3–18)	9 (3–17)	<0.001
Age at diagnosis (n, %)			<0.001
Pre-school age (≤6 years)	62 (13.1)	39 (28.5)	<0.001
Children (7–12 years)	232 (48.9)	78 (56.9)	0.121
Adolescent (13–18 years)	180 (38.0)	20 (14.6)	<0.001
Onset type (n, %)			<0.001
Acute (≤3 months)	65 (13.7)	43 (31.4)	<0.001
Acute recurrent (≤3 months)	189 (39.9)	19 (13.9)	<0.001
Chronic non-progressive (>3 months)	148 (31.2)	50 (36.5)	0.290
Chronic progressive (>3 months)	72 (15.2)	25 (18.2)	0.465
Localization (n, %)			<0.001
Diffuse	107 (22.6)	20 (14.6)	0.056
Localized	357 (75.3)	97 (70.8)	0.340
Mixed	10 (2.1)	20 (14.6)	<0.001
Duration (n, %)			0.289
<30 min	132 (27.9)	38 (27.7)	1.000
30–<60 min	93 (19.6)	35 (25.6)	0.167
≥1 h	249 (52.5)	64 (46.7)	0.270
Frequency (n, %)			<0.001
<2/month	60 (12.7)	0	<0.001
2–<4/month	96 (20.3)	49 (35.8)	<0.001
4–<15/month	146 (30.8)	50 (36.5)	0.249
≥15/month	67 (14.1)	38 (27.7)	<0.001
Daily	105 (22.1)	0	<0.001
Intensity (n, %)			<0.001
Mild	175 (36.9)	18 (13.1)	<0.001
Moderate	261 (55.1)	83 (60.6)	0.294
Severe	38 (8.0)	36 (26.3)	<0.001

Table 2. *Cont.*

Clinical Characteristics	TTH (n = 474)	HRS (n = 137)	*p*-Value
Sleep disturbance due to headache (n, %)	53 (11.2)	22 (16.1)	0.166
Morning headache (n, %)	113 (23.8)	33 (24.1)	1.000
Characteristics (n, %)			<0.001
Throbbing	21 (4.4)	34 (24.8)	<0.001
Sharp	1 (0.2)	9 (6.6)	<0.001
Cramping	3 (0.6)	1 (0.7)	1.000
Prickling	27 (5.7)	10 (7.3)	0.624
Constant/dull	83 (17.5)	10 (7.3)	0.005
Pressure	345 (72.8)	33 (24.1)	<0.001
Mixed	7 (1.5)	39 (28.5)	<0.001
Others	8 (1.7)	1 (0.7)	0.677
Accompanied symptoms (n, %)	168 (35.4)	78 (56.9)	<0.001
Nausea/vomiting	22 (4.6)	69 (50.4)	<0.001
Abdominal pain	15 (3.2)	15 (11.0)	<0.001
Photophobia	29 (6.1)	12 (8.8)	0.371
Phonophobia	43 (9.1)	0	<0.001
Dizziness	96 (20.3)	44 (32.1)	0.005
Nasal symptoms *	11 (2.3)	53 (38.7)	<0.001
Neurologic manifestations (n, %)	37 (7.8)	30 (21.9)	<0.001
Gait disturbance	0	2 (1.5)	0.074
Focal weakness	4 (0.8)	3 (2.2)	0.396
Visual disturbance	21 (4.4)	26 (19)	<0.001
Auditory symptoms #	1 (0.2)	10 (7.3)	<0.001
Dysarthria/aphasia	0	1 (0.7)	0.508
Dysesthesia	2 (0.4)	2 (1.5)	0.468
Decreased consciousness	5 (1.1)	2 (1.5)	1.000
Seizure	1 (0.2)	0	1.000
Movement symptom †	3 (0.6)	4 (2.9)	0.078
Triggering factors (n, %)	109 (23)	25 (18.2)	<0.001
Emotional stress	79 (16.6)	15 (11.0)	0.134
Hunger	0	0	-
Weather	15 (3.2)	2 (2.5)	0.439
Fatigue	24 (5.1)	15 (11.0)	0.022
Exercise	8 (1.7)	4 (2.9)	0.572
Light	0	2 (1.5)	0.074
Noise	2 (0.4)	0	1.000
Smell	8 (1.7)	0	0.270
Season at diagnosis (n, %)			0.458
Spring	107 (22.6)	35 (25.6)	0.541
Summer	133 (28.0)	45 (32.8)	0.327
Fall	125 (26.4)	30 (21.9)	0.343
Winger	109 (23.0)	27 (19.7)	0.485
Family history of migraine (n, %)	30 (6.8)	9 (6.6)	1.000
Family history of TTH (n, %)	114 (24.1)	3 (2.2)	<0.001
Family history of HRS (n, %)	5 (1.1)	36 (26.3)	<0.001
Family history of allergic rhinitis (n, %)	6 (1.3)	20 (14.6)	<0.001

† Tremor, myoclonus; * Rhinorrhea, nasal stuffiness, postnasal drip, snoring; # Ear fullness, tinnitus. TTH: tension-type headache, HRS: headache attributed to acute rhinosinusitis. *p*-values were derived using chi-square or Fisher's exact tests for categorical variables and Mann–Whitney U or *t*-tests for continuous variables, as appropriate.

3.2. Comparison Between HRS and Migraine

The HRS group was significantly younger at diagnosis compared with migraine (median: 9 vs. 12 years, interquartile range [IQR]: 6–11 vs. 9–14, $p < 0.001$) and exhibited a higher proportion of males (58.1% vs. 44.5%, $p < 0.001$). Preschool-aged children ($\leq$6 years) were markedly overrepresented in HRS (28.5% vs. 7.1%), whereas adolescents predominated in migraine (53.4% vs. 14.6%, both $p < 0.001$).

Headache onset patterns differed significantly ($p < 0.001$): acute onset (31.4%) and chronic non-progressive onset (44.5%) were more frequent in HRS, whereas chronic progressive onset was predominant in migraine (40.4%). Headache duration demonstrated distinct separation: short episodes (<1 h) were more common in HRS (41.6%), while migraine predominantly involved attacks lasting 4–72 h (74.8%, $p < 0.001$).

Headache frequency also differed ($p < 0.001$). HRS was characterized by 2–4 (35.8%) or 4–<15 (36.5%) episodes/month, with no daily headaches reported, whereas migraine exhibited higher daily headache prevalence (13.2%).

Accompanying symptoms were significantly more frequent in migraine (87.5% vs. 56.9%, $p < 0.001$), particularly nausea (74.2% vs. 50.4%), photophobia (68.9% vs. 19.7%), and phonophobia (58.1% vs. 0%). Neurologic manifestations were comparable in prevalence (25.1% vs. 21.9%, $p = 0.476$), but differed in distribution: migraine was associated with visual disturbances (19.6%), whereas HRS was more often linked to hearing impairment (7.3%). Triggering factors were reported by 23.3% of migraine and 18.2% of HRS patients ($p = 0.218$). The overall trigger distribution differed significantly ($p < 0.001$): fatigue was more frequent in HRS (11.0% vs. 4.8%), while migraine was more commonly associated with emotional stress and sensory stimuli, although individual differences did not reach statistical significance.

Pain localization (Figure 1) also differed: temporal (62.3% vs. 49.6%) and parietal pain (33.6% vs. 21.9%) were more common in migraine, whereas vertex (15.3% vs. 6.1%) and occipital pain (12.4% vs. 4.9%) were more frequent in HRS (all $p < 0.05$). Laterality further distinguished groups: unilateral pain predominated in migraine (66.8%), whereas HRS displayed a mixed pattern (49.8% bilateral, 42.3% unilateral, $p < 0.001$).

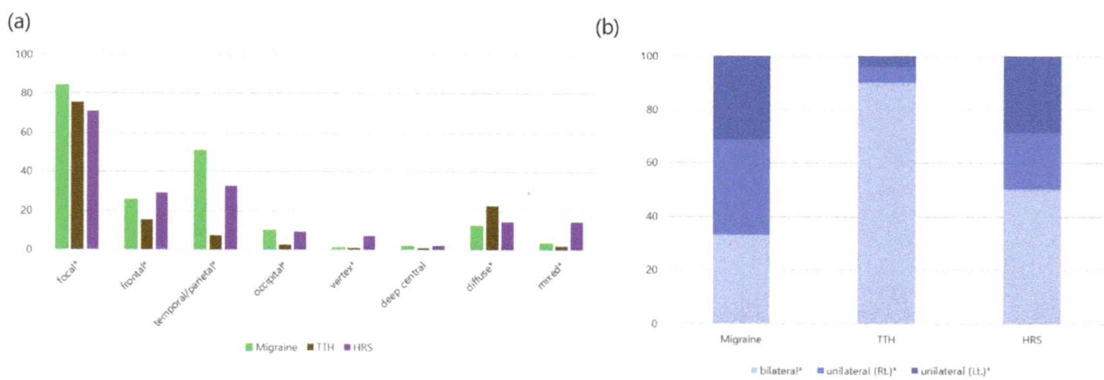

Figure 1. (**a**) Comparison of headache pain locations among patients with migraine, TTH, and HRS. (**b**) Comparison of headache laterality among patients with migraine, TTH, and HRS. Stacked bar graphs show the distribution of bilateral and unilateral (right or left) headache presentations in each group. Asterisks (*) indicate significant differences. Bar graphs display mean ± SD (%) of localization and laterality.

The HRS group showed several distinctive features compared with migraine:

- Younger age at diagnosis (median 9 vs. 12 years, $p < 0.001$).
- Higher proportion of males (58.1% vs. 44.5%, $p < 0.001$).
- More preschool-age patients (28.5% vs. 7.1%, $p < 0.001$).
- Shorter headache duration (<1 h: 41.6% vs. 12.8%, $p < 0.001$).
- Fewer sensory symptoms such as photophobia and phonophobia, but more nasal and auditory symptoms ($p < 0.001$).

3.3. Comparison Between HRS and TTH

HRS patients were significantly younger than those with TTH (median: 9 vs. 11 years, interquartile range [IQR]: 6–11 vs. 8–14, $p < 0.001$) and more frequently male (58.1% vs. 48.9%, $p = 0.035$). Preschool-aged children (≤6 years) were markedly overrepresented in HRS (28.5% vs. 13.1%), whereas adolescents predominated in TTH (38.0% vs. 14.6%, both $p < 0.001$).

Headache onset patterns differed significantly ($p < 0.001$). Acute onset was more common in HRS (31.4% vs. 13.7%), while acute recurrent onset characterized TTH (39.9% vs. 13.9%). Chronic non-progressive onset was observed more often in HRS (36.5% vs. 31.2%), while chronic progressive onset frequencies were comparable (18.2% vs. 15.2%). Headache intensity and pain characteristics showed marked differences. Severe pain was more frequent in HRS (26.3% vs. 8.0%, $p < 0.001$), while mild pain predominated in TTH (36.9% vs. 13.1%, $p < 0.001$). Pressure-type pain (72.8% vs. 24.1%, $p < 0.001$) and constant/dull pain (17.5% vs. 7.3%, $p = 0.005$) were typical of TTH, whereas throbbing (24.8% vs. 4.4%, $p < 0.001$) and mixed pain (28.5% vs. 1.5%, $p < 0.001$) were enriched in HRS.

Accompanying symptoms were more prevalent in HRS (56.9% vs. 35.4%, $p < 0.001$), including nausea/vomiting (50.4% vs. 4.6%), abdominal pain (11.0% vs. 3.2%), dizziness (32.1% vs. 20.3%), and nasal symptoms (38.7% vs. 2.3%). Neurologic manifestations were significantly higher in HRS (21.9% vs. 7.8%, $p < 0.001$), with visual disturbances (19.0% vs. 4.4%) and hearing impairment (7.3% vs. 0.2%) particularly notable. Triggering factors were less frequent overall but differed in pattern ($p < 0.001$): fatigue was more common in HRS (11.0% vs. 5.1%), whereas emotional stress predominated in TTH (16.6% vs. 11.0%).

Family history also revealed distinct associations: allergic rhinitis (14.6% vs. 1.3%) and HRS (26.3% vs. 1.1%) were enriched in HRS, whereas familial TTH was more frequent in TTH (24.1% vs. 2.2%, all $p < 0.001$). Notably, migraine family history rates were low and comparable (6.8% vs. 6.6%).

The key differences between HRS and TTH can be summarized as follows:

- Younger age at diagnosis in HRS (median 9 vs. 11 years, $p < 0.001$).
- Higher proportion of males (58.1% vs. 48.9%, $p < 0.001$).
- More preschool-age patients and fewer adolescents ($p < 0.001$).
- Greater headache intensity and more nasal/auditory symptoms ($p < 0.001$).
- Less frequent fatigue as a trigger ($p = 0.045$).

3.4. Symptom Profiling and Cluster Analysis

Principal component analysis (PCA) of 12 headache-related symptoms demonstrated that the first two components (PC1 and PC2) accounted for 10.9% and 9.4% of the total variance, respectively (Figure 2). In the PCA plot, PC1 mainly reflected sensory hypersensitivity symptoms such as photophobia, phonophobia, and nausea, while PC2 represented sinonasal and otologic features including nasal congestion and hearing impairment. Migraine cases tended to cluster along PC1, HRS along PC2, and TTH showed wide overlap between both axes. These distributions indicate partial separation but substantial overlap among headache subtypes. Migraine cases partially aggregated along PC1, largely driven by sensory hypersensitivity features such as photophobia, phonophobia, and nausea, whereas HRS aligned predominantly along PC2 due to sinonasal symptoms, hearing impairment, and fatigue. TTH exhibited diffuse distribution across both axes, reflecting its overlap with non-specific symptoms. Despite partial aggregation, substantial intergroup overlap was evident, underscoring phenotypic heterogeneity across diagnoses. K-means clustering identified three symptom-based clusters: (1) migraine-dominant with sensory hypersensitivity (photophobia, phonophobia, nausea), (2) HRS-dominant with sinonasal and otologic features (nasal congestion, rhinorrhea, hearing impairment), and (3) mixed profiles characterized by dizziness and fatigue irrespective of diagnosis. Notably, each cluster contained cases from multiple diagnostic categories, highlighting that symptom combinations transcend conventional diagnostic boundaries.

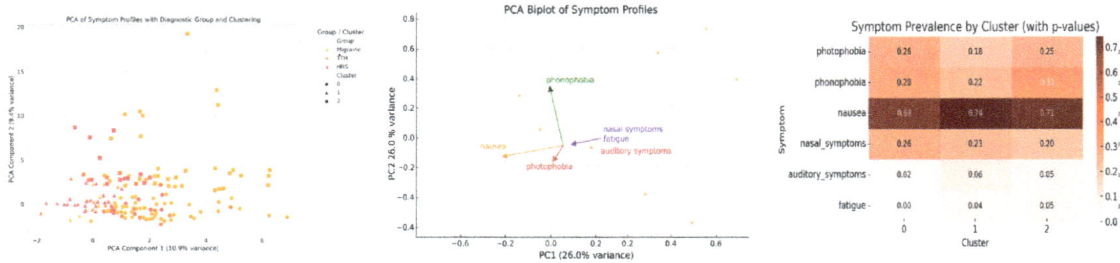

(a) (b) (c)

Figure 2. Multivariate symptom profiling across headache subtypes. PCA revealed partial but distinct separation among migraine, TTH, and HRS (**a**). The biplot identified sensory hypersensitivity versus sinonasal–otologic features as the main differentiating axes (**b**). × = individual patient scores; arrows = symptom loadings. Cluster-based heatmap confirmed that nasal and auditory symptoms were predominant in the HRS-dominant cluster (**c**).

3.5. Supplementary Table S1: Three-Group Comparison

Supplementary Table S1 compares migraine, TTH, and HRS across demographic and clinical variables. Age distribution differed significantly ($p < 0.001$): HRS was enriched in preschool-aged children (28.5%), TTH in school-aged children (48.9%), and migraine in adolescents (53.4%). Headache onset patterns varied ($p < 0.001$), with acute and chronic non-progressive onset predominating in HRS, chronic progressive onset in migraine, and acute recurrent onset in TTH. Headache localization differed markedly ($p < 0.001$): focal pain was most frequent in migraine (83.9%), while diffuse pain was more common in TTH (22.6%) and mixed pain in HRS (14.6%). Laterality also showed clear separation ($p < 0.001$): unilateral pain predominated in migraine (66.8%), bilateral pain in TTH (90.0%), and HRS exhibited an intermediate distribution (50.2% bilateral, 42.3% unilateral).

Accompanying symptoms were significantly more prevalent in migraine and HRS compared to TTH, including nausea/vomiting (74.2%, 50.4% vs. 4.6%) and dizziness (34.6%, 32.1% vs. 20.3%). Nasal symptoms were unique to HRS (38.7%, $p < 0.001$). Neurologic manifestations followed a gradient: migraine (25.1%) > HRS (21.9%) > TTH (7.8%). Triggering factors differed significantly ($p < 0.001$): fatigue was most associated with HRS (11.0%), while emotional stress predominated in TTH (16.6%). Family history patterns showed diagnosis-specific clustering: migraine was strongly linked to familial migraine (32.9%), TTH to familial TTH (24.1%), and HRS to allergic rhinitis (14.6%) and familial HRS (26.3%). These findings reinforce distinct demographic and phenotypic profiles while highlighting overlapping features that complicate diagnosis.

3.6. Multivariate Predictors of HRS

Multivariate logistic regression (Table 3) identified several independent predictors of HRS. Younger age (OR = 0.71, 95% CI: 0.522–0.967, $p = 0.030$) and male sex (OR = 0.567, 95% CI: 0.334–0.963, $p = 0.036$) were inversely associated with HRS, indicating that younger boys were more likely to be diagnosed with HRS. Shorter headache duration (OR = 0.62, 95% CI: 0.484–0.793, $p < 0.001$) and higher pain intensity (OR = 2.165, 95% CI: 1.380–3.397, $p = 0.001$) were also significant predictors. Otolaryngologic and allergic features showed the strongest associations: nasal symptoms (OR = 9.836, 95% CI: 4.548–21.273), hearing impairment (OR = 22.52, 95% CI: 7.153–70.989), family history of HRS (OR = 32.602, 95% CI: 14.312–74.265), and allergic rhinitis (OR = 8.468, 95% CI: 3.484–20.582) were all highly predictive (all $p < 0.001$). Fatigue also emerged as an independent predictor (OR = 3.935, 95% CI: 1.715–9.029, $p = 0.001$).

Table 3. Multivariate analysis of predictive factors for HRS.

Factors	OR	95% CI	*p*-Value
Male sex	0.567	0.334–0.963	0.036
Age	0.71	0.522–0.967	0.030
Location	1.57	0.794–3.102	0.194
Duration	0.62	0.484–0.793	<0.001
Frequency	1.217	0.988–1.499	0.065
Intensity	2.165	1.380–3.397	0.001
Nausea/vomiting	1.046	0.609–1.796	0.870
Photophobia	0.412	0.145–1.172	0.097
Phonophobia	0.398	0.123–1.165	0.998
Nasal symptoms	9.836	4.548–21.273	<0.001
Auditory symptoms	22.52	7.153–70.989	<0.001
Fatigue	3.935	1.715–9.029	0.001
Family history of HRS	32.602	14.312–74.265	<0.001
Family history of allergic rhinitis	8.468	3.484–20.582	<0.001

HRS: headache attributed to acute rhinosinusitis, OR: odds ratio, CI: confidence interval. The chi-square test or Fisher's exact test (for small cell counts) was used for categorical comparisons.

In contrast, headache frequency (OR = 1.217, $p = 0.065$), pain location (OR = 1.57, $p = 0.194$), nausea/vomiting (OR = 1.046, $p = 0.870$), photophobia (OR = 0.412, $p = 0.097$), and phonophobia (OR = 0.398, $p = 0.998$) were not independently associated with HRS in the multivariate model.

4. Discussion

This study comprehensively compared migraine, TTH, and HRS in a large pediatric cohort, highlighting both shared and distinguishing features. We also identified independent predictive factors for HRS using multivariate analysis, offering clinically relevant tools to improve diagnostic accuracy and inform tailored management strategies in children and adolescents.

4.1. Comparison with Previous Studies

Our findings reaffirm prior reports that HRS is more common in younger children and characterized by acute onset, shorter headache duration, and otolaryngologic symptoms such as nasal congestion and rhinorrhea [11,13,16]. In contrast, migraine predominated in adolescents and was associated with longer attack duration, higher frequency, and migrainous features—including throbbing pain, photophobia, phonophobia, and nausea—consistent with its established diagnostic criteria [9]. TTH displayed the expected phenotype of bilateral, pressing-type pain with fewer associated symptoms, aligning with its musculoskeletal pathophysiology [17,18]. The key distinguishing clinical features among migraine, tension-type headache, and headache attributed to rhinosinusitis are summarized in Supplementary Table S2.

However, our study diverges from earlier literature in several respects. Prior studies have linked migraine occurrence to seasonal peaks in winter or spring [19,20] and HRS to allergy-associated seasons [12,21], In contrast, we observed no significant seasonal variation across diagnostic groups, with peak case numbers occurring during summer months. This discrepancy may reflect regional climatic differences, relatively stable allergen exposure patterns, or sociobehavioral factors such as school calendar-related stress or healthcare utilization unique to our population [22]. historical clinical markers such as early-morning headaches or sleep-disrupting pain, which have been proposed to distinguish secondary from primary headaches [11,23], were not discriminative in our cohort. This finding suggests that such features may be less reliable in modern practice, where early neuroimaging, routine otolaryngologic assessment, and broader access to pediatric headache specialists reduce reliance on indirect or historical diagnostic cues.

4.2. HRS Versus Primary Headaches: Shared and Distinguishing Features

Notably, 27.7% of HRS patients in our cohort were initially misclassified as primary headache (migraine or TTH), underscoring the substantial clinical overlap and diagnostic challenge, particularly in younger children with limited ability to describe sensory features. This finding is consistent with prior studies reporting that 42–80% of patients initially labeled as 'sinus headache' were ultimately diagnosed with migraine following specialist evaluation [17,24]. These data highlight the importance of incorporating sinonasal findings—such as nasal symptoms or hearing impairment—into diagnostic pathways to improve diagnostic accuracy.

Although HRS exhibited distinct features, it also shared several characteristics with migraine and TTH. Neurologic manifestations were unexpectedly frequent in HRS (21.9%), second only to migraine (25.1%), and higher than previously reported [25]. While visual disturbances predominated in migraines, HRS was more often associated with hearing impairment and dizziness. This may be attributable to sinus inflammation and its anatomical proximity to cranial nerves, referred pain mechanisms, or secondary venous congestion [26,27]. Moreover, overlapping autonomic features—such as nasal congestion and rhinorrhea—may arise from shared trigeminovascular activation, further obscuring the boundary between HRS and migraine and contributing to frequent misdiagnosis in both pediatric and adult populations [24,28]. This overlap is especially problematic in young children who cannot reliably articulate sensory or autonomic symptoms, emphasizing the diagnostic value of caregiver reports and comprehensive otolaryngologic assessment.

Pain topography further revealed differentiating clues: temporal and parietal pain were common to both migraine and HRS, whereas vertex and occipital pain were significantly enriched in HRS, consistent with posterior paranasal sinus involvement [29–31]. Headache laterality also varied: unilateral pain predominated in migraine, bilateral pain in TTH, while HRS displayed an intermediate mixed pattern [4,32]. These anatomical distinctions may assist differentiation, especially in diagnostically ambiguous cases. Emerging evidence suggests that sinus inflammation in HRS can activate trigeminal nociceptive pathways and perivascular meningeal afferents, resulting in pain patterns that closely mimic migraine. Pro-inflammatory cytokines such as interleukin-6 and tumor necrosis factor-alpha, detected in acute bacterial sinusitis, may sensitize trigeminovascular circuits [33]. Additionally, venous congestion in the cavernous sinus and perisinusoidal regions may produce referred orbital and frontal pain frequently mistaken for migraine [34]. This neuroinflammatory overlap underscores the neurovascular interface linking HRS and migraine and reinforces the need for timely otolaryngology referral and targeted evaluation in diagnostically ambiguous cases.

4.3. Clinical Implications and Application of Predictors

While radiologic sinus changes support HRS diagnosis, their non-specificity limits their standalone utility, as incidental sinus opacification is observed in up to 30% of asymptomatic children undergoing brain MRI [35]. Incorporating nasal endoscopy, when feasible, may enhance diagnostic confidence by allowing direct visualization of purulent drainage or mucosal edema [36]. Additionally, validated pediatric sinonasal symptom scales, such as the SN-5 (Sinus and Nasal Quality of Life Survey), can complement headache evaluation by quantifying sinonasal symptom burden and improving diagnostic accuracy [37].

Incorporating the clinical predictors identified in our multivariate analysis—namely, younger age, male sex, shorter headache duration, high pain intensity, nasal symptoms, hearing impairment, fatigue, family history of HRS, and allergic rhinitis—into routine assessment may significantly improve diagnostic precision. These findings align with existing literature linking allergic sensitization and otolaryngologic pathology to HRS [13,21]. For example, a preschool-aged child presenting with acute, severe headache, nasal congestion, and a positive family history of allergic rhinitis should prompt early otolaryngologic referral and consideration of HRS, even in the absence of typical migraine features.

Clinically, these predictors provide a pragmatic framework for triaging pediatric headache patients, reducing reliance on neuroimaging, and avoiding delays in appropriate treatment. Comprehensive nasal and otolaryngologic examination, coupled with systematic inquiry into allergic and familial history, can facilitate early identification of HRS and enable targeted interventions such as antibiotics, decongestants, or allergy management rather than empiric migraine therapy. Based on these independent predictors, a simplified diagnostic algorithm for pediatric headache attributed to rhinosinusitis was developed to assist clinical decision-making (Supplementary Figure S1)

Integrating these predictors into structured triage algorithms may also optimize healthcare resource utilization. Early recognition of HRS can decrease unnecessary neuroimaging, reduce inappropriate migraine pharmacotherapy, and expedite appropriate antibiotic or decongestant initiation. Prior cost-effectiveness analyses support that otolaryngology referral pathways incorporating symptom-based screening can reduce diagnostic delays by 30–40% while lowering imaging costs [38].

Given these diagnostic challenges, clinicians should adopt structured approaches that integrate headache phenotype, otolaryngologic features, allergic/familial history, and environmental context. While prior studies have emphasized triggers such as weather or barometric pressure changes in migraine [39], our cohort demonstrated low rates of weather-related triggers but a strong association with fatigue, highlighting the need for population-specific trigger profiling [40]. Standardized screening tools, including pediatric migraine trigger questionnaires, may further enhance history-taking and contextualize headache triggers across subtypes.

In younger children, limited ability to verbalize headache quality or associated symptoms necessitates greater reliance on caregiver observations, otolaryngologic examination, and indirect behavioral cues. Signs such as irritability, disrupted sleep, or facial tenderness on palpation may serve as surrogate markers of sinus-related pain in non-verbal or preschool-aged patients. Our finding that 28.5% of HRS cases occurred in preschool-aged children underscores the need for age-tailored assessment frameworks and early otolaryngologic involvement in this group.

4.4. Integration with Existing Literature

Our findings are consistent with reports highlighting the phenotypic heterogeneity of pediatric headache. Previous studies have reported that 40–60% of pediatric migraine cases are initially misdiagnosed as sinusitis, leading to delayed or inappropriate treatment [26]. PCA and clustering analyses revealed significant overlap between diagnoses, explaining only modest variance (10.9% and 9.4%), supporting the concept of a clinical continuum rather than discrete entities [41,42]. This aligns with emerging machine learning studies advocating for multidimensional classification systems that transcend traditional ICHD criteria. Such models may better capture intermediate phenotypes such as HRS-migraine overlap, facilitating tailored management strategies.

Furthermore, the relatively high rate of neurologic symptoms in HRS suggests that clinicians should not dismiss transient sensory or visual disturbances in the context of suspected sinus-related headache. Rather, these should prompt careful evaluation for otolaryngologic pathology in conjunction with neurologic work-up, avoiding premature assignment to primary headache categories [12,39].

4.5. Limitations and Future Directions

Integrating multivariate predictors into predictive nomograms or electronic clinical decision-support tools has the potential to standardize diagnosis across both primary and specialty care. Machine learning approaches—such as random forest and gradient boosting models that incorporate symptom clusters, allergy history, and demographic variables—have shown promise in pediatric headache classification and could be leveraged to further refine HRS detection [43].

This study has several limitations. First, its retrospective design introduces inherent documentation bias, particularly for subjective features such as photophobia, headache timing, and pain descriptors, which may be underreported or inconsistently recorded. Second, otolaryngologic findings were derived primarily from radiology reports rather than validated sinus scoring systems, limiting the granularity of sinonasal assessment. Third, our clustering and PCA analyses were exploratory in nature and accounted for only modest variance, underscoring the need for validation in larger, prospective cohorts. Finally, because our data were derived from a tertiary-care setting, generalizability to primary care or community populations may be limited. Information on medication use was unavailable in our retrospective dataset; therefore, potential similarities in drug response between HRS and migraine could not be evaluated and were noted as a limitation. It should also be noted that sinus-related and primary headaches may coexist in the same patient, and their clinical features can overlap; thus, complete differentiation is not always possible in clinical practice.

Another potential concern is the selection of patients, as most participants were recruited from tertiary pediatric neurology clinics. In the United States and other Western healthcare systems, children with acute headache symptoms are often first evaluated in primary care or emergency settings, and referral to pediatric neurology may be delayed. However, in Korea, patients and caregivers can directly access tertiary centers without requiring primary care referral, and acute headache presentations are commonly seen in pediatric neurology clinics. Thus, our cohort reflects the actual referral patterns in the Korean healthcare system, which should be considered when interpreting the generalizability of our findings.

Future studies should be prospective and multicentric, incorporating standardized allergy testing, validated otolaryngologic scoring systems (e.g., Lund-Mackay or SN-5), and longitudinal headache diaries to improve phenotypic resolution. Additionally, integration of advanced analytical methods, including machine learning algorithms and multi-omics approaches (e.g., transcriptomic or cytokine profiling), could facilitate a mechanistic understanding of the overlap between HRS and primary headaches and enable the development of personalized, phenotype-driven diagnostic frameworks.

5. Conclusions

This study identified key clinical predictors that distinguish pediatric headache attributed to rhinosinusitis (HRS) from migraine and tension-type headache. Younger age, male sex, short headache duration, high pain intensity, nasal and auditory symptoms, allergic rhinitis, and family history of HRS were the most reliable indicators. Integrating these predictors into clinical evaluation may reduce misdiagnosis, limit unnecessary neuroimaging, and guide timely otolaryngologic referral. Future multicenter prospective studies using standardized sinonasal scoring and machine-learning–based models are warranted to refine diagnostic algorithms for pediatric HRS.

Supplementary Materials: The following supporting information can be downloaded at: https://www.mdpi.com/article/10.3390/children12111557/s1, Table S1: Comparison of headache characteristics between the migraine, TTH and HRS. Table S2: Clinical differences between migraine, TTH, and HRS. Figure S1: Clinical diagnostic algorithm for pediatric HRS.

Author Contributions: Conceptualization, S.B.H. and J.Y.H.; methodology, E.G.P.; software, E.G.P.; validation, E.G.P., S.B.H. and J.Y.H.; formal analysis, S.B.H.; investigation, S.B.H.; resources, E.G.P.; data curation, S.B.H.; writing—original draft preparation, S.B.H.; writing—review and editing, J.Y.H.; visualization, E.G.P.; supervision, J.Y.H.; project administration, J.Y.H.; funding acquisition, E.G.P. All authors have read and agreed to the published version of the manuscript.

Funding: This study received no specific grant from any funding agency in the public, commercial, or not-for-profit sectors.

Institutional Review Board Statement: This study was conducted in accordance with the principles of the Declaration of Helsinki. The study protocol was reviewed and approved by the IRB of the Catholic Medical Center (approval numbers: OC23RASI0159, approved on 7 September 2024; and DC24RASI0047, approved on 7 June 2024). The requirement for informed consent was waived due to the retrospective design and the use of anonymized data.

Informed Consent Statement: Patient consent was waived due to the retrospective nature of the study and the use of anonymized data, as approved by the IRB.

Data Availability Statement: The data that support the findings of this study are not publicly available due to ethical and privacy restrictions involving pediatric patient records. However, de-identified data may be available from the corresponding author upon reasonable request and with appropriate IRB approval.

Acknowledgments: The authors thank the pediatric neurology and otolaryngology teams at Daejeon, Incheon, and Bucheon St. Mary's Hospitals for their assistance with patient recruitment and data collection. We also thank the biostatistics support team for their valuable advice on data analysis.

Conflicts of Interest: The authors declare that there are no potential conflicts of interest with respect to the research, authorship, or publication of this article.

Abbreviations

The following abbreviations are used in this manuscript:

HRS	Headache attributed to rhinosinusitis
TTH	Tension-type headache
OR	Odds ratio
CL	Confidence interval
PC	Principal component
ROC	Receiver operating characteristics
ICHD	International classification of headache disorders
IRB	Institutional review board

References

1. Mehle, M.E. What Do We Know about Rhinogenic Headache? The otolaryngologist's challenge. *Otolaryngol. Clin. N. Am.* **2014**, *47*, 255–268. [CrossRef]
2. Lewis, D.; Ashwal, S.; Dahl, G.; Dorbad, D.; Hirtz, D.; Prensky, A.; Jarjour, I. Practice Parameter: Evaluation of Children and Adolescents with Recurrent Headaches: Report of the Quality Standards Subcommittee of the American Academy of Neurology and the Practice Committee of the Child Neurology Society. *Neurology* **2002**, *59*, 490–498. [CrossRef]
3. Iseh, K.; Makusidi, M. Rhinosinusitis: A Retrospective Analysis of Clinical Pattern and Outcome in North Western Nigeria. *Ann. Afr. Med.* **2010**, *9*, 20–26. [CrossRef]
4. Şenbil, N.; Gurer, Y.K.; Arslan, D.; Barlas, O.; Deda, G. Sinusitis in Children and Adolescents with Chronic or Recurrent Headache: A Case–Control Study. *J. Headache Pain* **2008**, *9*, 33–36. [CrossRef]
5. Hu, S.; Wu, J.; Liu, J.; Xu, G.; Gu, M. The Role of the Otolaryngologist in the Evaluation and Management of Headaches. *Am. J. Otolaryngol.* **2019**, *40*, 115–120. [CrossRef]
6. Abu-Arafeh, I.; Razak, S.; Sivaraman, B.; Graham, C. Prevalence of Headache and Migraine in Children and Adolescents: A Systematic Review of Population-Based Studies. *Dev. Med. Child Neurol.* **2010**, *52*, 1088–1097. [CrossRef]
7. Schreiber, C.P.; Hutchinson, S.; Webster, C.J.; Ames, M.; Richardson, M.S.; Powers, C. Prevalence of Migraine in Patients with a History of Self-Reported or Physician-Diagnosed "Sinus" Headache. *Arch. Intern. Med.* **2004**, *164*, 1769–1772. [CrossRef] [PubMed]
8. Onofri, A.; Chisari, C.; Martelletti, P. Primary Headache Epidemiology in Children and Adolescents: A Systematic Review and Meta-Analysis. *J. Headache Pain* **2023**, *24*, 8. [CrossRef] [PubMed]
9. Arnold, M.; Headache Classification Committee of the International Headache Society (IHS). The International Classification of Headache Disorders, 3rd Edition. *Cephalalgia* **2018**, *38*, 1–211. [CrossRef] [PubMed]
10. Patel, Z.M.; Setzen, M.; Poetker, D.M.; DelGaudio, J.M. "Sinus Headache": Rhinogenic Headache or Migraine? An Evidence-Based Guide to Diagnosis and Treatment. *Int. Forum Allergy Rhinol.* **2013**, *3*, 221–230. [CrossRef]
11. Eross, E.; Dodick, D.; Eross, M. The Sinus, Allergy and Migraine Study (SAMS). *Headache* **2007**, *47*, 213–224. [CrossRef]
12. Ceriani, C.E.; Silberstein, S.D. Headache and Rhinosinusitis: A Review. *Cephalalgia* **2021**, *41*, 453–463. [CrossRef]
13. Smith, B.C.; Adappa, N.D.; Palmer, J.N.; Kennedy, D.W.; Chiu, A.G. Rhinogenic Headache in Pediatric and Adolescent Patients: An Evidence-Based Review. *Int. Forum Allergy Rhinol.* **2019**, *9*, 511–517. [CrossRef]
14. Khan, A.; Liu, S.; Tao, F. Current Trends in Pediatric Migraine: Clinical Insights and Therapeutic Strategies. *Brain Sci.* **2025**, *15*, 280. [CrossRef] [PubMed]
15. Bellini, B.; Arruda, M.; Cescut, A.; Saulle, C.; Persico, A.; Carotenuto, M.; Gatta, M.; Nacinovich, R.; Piazza, F.; Termine, C. Headache and Comorbidity in Children and Adolescents. *J. Headache Pain* **2013**, *14*, 79. [CrossRef] [PubMed]
16. Greene, K.; Irwin, S.L.; Gelfand, A.A. Pediatric Migraine: An Update. *Neurol. Clin.* **2019**, *37*, 815–833. [CrossRef] [PubMed]
17. Jones, N.S. Sinus Headaches: Avoiding Over- and Mis-Diagnosis. *Expert Rev. Neurother.* **2009**, *9*, 439–444. [CrossRef]
18. Poulsen, A.H.; Kjaergaard, A.D.; Hansen, T.F.; Olesen, J. The Chronobiology of Migraine: A Systematic Review. *J. Headache Pain* **2021**, *22*, 76. [CrossRef]
19. Alstadhaug, K.; Salvesen, R.; Bekkelund, S. Seasonal Variation in Migraine. *Cephalalgia* **2005**, *25*, 811–816. [CrossRef]
20. Soriani, S.; Fiumana, E.; Manfredini, R.; Boari, B.; Scalas, C.; Battistella, P.A. Circadian and Seasonal Variation of Migraine Attacks in Children. *Headache* **2006**, *46*, 1571–1574. [CrossRef]
21. Tang, S.J.; Lin, C.W.; Huang, C.Y.; Hsieh, Y.L.; Lin, Y.C. A Comparison of Clinical Features of Youth with and without Rhinitis Signs and Symptoms Who Are Hospitalized for Headache. *Children* **2022**, *9*, 1241. [CrossRef]
22. Kröner-Herwig, B.; Gassmann, J. Headache Disorders in Children and Adolescents: Their Association with Psychological, Behavioral, and Socio-Environmental Factors. *Headache* **2012**, *52*, 1387–1401. [CrossRef]

23. Bigal, M.E.; Lipton, R.B. The Differential Diagnosis of Chronic Daily Headaches: An Algorithm-Based Approach. *J. Headache Pain* **2007**, *8*, 263–272. [CrossRef]
24. Robblee, J.; Secora, K.A. Debunking Myths: Sinus Headache. *Curr. Neurol. Neurosci. Rep.* **2021**, *21*, 42. [CrossRef] [PubMed]
25. Kaur, A.; Singh, A. Clinical Study of Headache in Relation to Sinusitis and Its Management. *J. Med. Life* **2013**, *6*, 389–392. [PubMed]
26. Park, E.G.; Kim, J.Y.; Lee, J.Y.; Han, J.Y. Headache Attributed to Rhinosinusitis in Pediatric Patients: Clinical Insights and Diagnostic Implications. *Transl. Pediatr.* **2025**, *14*, 161–170. [CrossRef]
27. Mustafa, M.; Patawari, P.; Iftikhar, H.M.; Shimmi, S.C.; Hussain, S.S.; Sein, M.M. Acute and chronic rhinosinusitis: Pathophysiology and treatment. *Int. J. Pharm. Sci. Invent.* **2015**, *4*, 30–36.
28. Cady, R.K.; Schreiber, C.P. Sinus Headache or Migraine? Considerations in Making a Differential Diagnosis. *Neurology* **2002**, *58*, S10–S14. [CrossRef]
29. Loder, E.; Weizenbaum, E.; Giddon, D. Migraine Pain Location and Measures of Healthcare Use and Distress: An Observational Study. *Pain Res. Manag.* **2018**, *2018*, 6157982. [CrossRef]
30. Brna, P.M.; Dooley, J.M. Headaches in the Pediatric Population. *Semin. Pediatr. Neurol.* **2006**, *13*, 222–230. [CrossRef]
31. Ramadan, H.H.; Chaiban, R.; Makary, C. Pediatric Rhinosinusitis. *Pediatr. Clin. N. Am.* **2022**, *69*, 275–286. [CrossRef]
32. Karlı, N.; Akyol, A.; Uçler, S.; Baykan, B.; Zarifoğlu, M.; Siva, A.; Saip, S.; Ertaş, M.; Oğuz, H.; Özge, A. Clinical Characteristics of Tension-Type Headache and Migraine in Adolescents: A Student-Based Study. *Headache* **2006**, *46*, 399–412. [CrossRef]
33. Fokkens, W.J.; Lund, V.J.; Hopkins, C.; Hellings, P.W.; Kern, R.; Reitsma, S.; Toppila-Salmi, S.; Bernal-Sprekelsen, M.; Mullol, J.; Alobid, I.; et al. European Position Paper on Rhinosinusitis and Nasal Polyps 2020. *Rhinology* **2020**, *58* (Suppl. S29), 1–464. [CrossRef]
34. Godley, F.A.; O'Brien, E.K.; Orlandi, R.R.; Smith, T.L.; Soler, Z.M. Update on the Diagnostic Considerations for Neurogenic Nasal and Sinus Symptoms: A Current Review Suggests Adding a Possible Diagnosis of Migraine. *Am. J. Otolaryngol.* **2019**, *40*, 306–311. [CrossRef] [PubMed]
35. Von Kalle, T.; Kaiser, W.A.; Mentzel, H.J. Incidental Findings in Paranasal Sinuses and Mastoid Cells: A Cross-Sectional Magnetic Resonance Imaging (MRI) Study in a Pediatric Radiology Department. *RoFo* **2012**, *184*, 629–634. [CrossRef] [PubMed]
36. Peters, A.T.; Spector, S.; Hsu, J.; Baroody, F.M.; Chandra, R.K.; Grammer, L.C.; Kennedy, D.W.; Cohen, N.A.; Kaliner, M.A.; Wald, E.R.; et al. Diagnosis and Management of Rhinosinusitis: A Practice Parameter Update. *Ann. Allergy Asthma Immunol.* **2014**, *113*, 347–385. [CrossRef]
37. Kay, D.J.; Rosenfeld, R.M. Quality of Life for Children with Persistent Sinonasal Symptoms. *Otolaryngol. Head Neck Surg.* **2003**, *128*, 17–26. [CrossRef] [PubMed]
38. Leung, R.M.; Smith, T.L.; Rudmik, L.; Mace, J.C.; Smith, S.B.; Schlosser, R.J.; Soler, Z.M. Primary Care and Upfront Computed Tomography Scanning in the Diagnosis of Chronic Rhinosinusitis: A Cost-Based Decision Analysis. *Laryngoscope* **2014**, *124*, 12–18. [CrossRef]
39. Park, J.W.; Cho, S.J.; Chu, M.K. Analysis of Trigger Factors in Episodic Migraineurs Using a Smartphone Headache Diary Application. *PLoS ONE* **2016**, *11*, e0149577. [CrossRef]
40. Son, H.J.; Jin, J.O.; Lee, K.H. Evaluation of Pediatric Migraine Triggers: A Single-Center Study. *Clin. Exp. Pediatr.* **2024**, *68*, 163–170. [CrossRef]
41. Radziwon, J.; Waszak, P. Seasonal Changes of Internet Searching Suggest Circannual Rhythmicity of Primary Headache Disorders. *Headache* **2022**, *62*, 811–817. [CrossRef] [PubMed]
42. Baglioni, V.; D'Acunto, G.; Balestri, M.; Maestri, M.; Pochiero, G.; Zamponi, N.; Bravaccio, C.; Termine, C.; Cecchini, A.P.; Sansone, M.; et al. Tension-Type Headache in Children and Adolescents. *Life* **2023**, *13*, 825. [CrossRef] [PubMed]
43. Stubberud, A.; Alstadhaug, K.B.; Sand, T. Artificial Intelligence and Headache. *Cephalalgia* **2024**, *44*, 03331024241268290. [CrossRef] [PubMed]

children

MDPI

Article

Training, Awareness, and Clinical Perspectives of Pediatric Dentists on Headache and Migraine Management: A National Survey Study

Samantha Glover [1], Linda Sangalli [2] and Caroline M. Sawicki [1,*]

1 Department of Pediatric Dentistry and Dental Public Health, University of North Carolina, Chapel Hill, NC 27599, USA; sag40@email.unc.edu
2 College of Dental Medicine—Illinois, Midwestern University, Downers Grove, IL 60515, USA; lsanga@midwestern.edu
* Correspondence: caroline_sawicki@unc.edu

Abstract

Background/Objectives: Migraine affects approximately 3–10% of school-aged children and up to 28% of adolescents, with prevalence increasing during adolescence. For pediatric specialty providers, increased awareness of this condition may influence patient care. This study examined pediatric dentists' education, clinical exposure, and perceived knowledge gaps related to pediatric migraine, with the goal of identifying barriers to recognition and referral, as well as informing future training to support accurate diagnosis and interdisciplinary care. **Methods:** A 28-item electronic questionnaire was distributed to all members of the American Academy of Pediatric Dentistry, including pediatric dentists and postgraduate pediatric dental residents, assessing knowledge, beliefs, clinical experience, and interest in further training regarding pediatric headache/migraine management. Respondents with and without previous training were compared in terms of general understanding using *t*-tests; a linear regression model analyzed predictors of provider awareness regarding links between oral conditions and headache/migraine. **Results:** Among 315 respondents, the mean self-perceived awareness score was 2.7 ± 1.3 (on a 0–5 scale). The most frequently identified contributing factors were clenching (73.7%), bruxism (72.4%), and temporomandibular disorders (65.7%). Nearly all respondents (95.2%) reported no formal education on headache/migraine prevention, yet 78.1% agreed on the importance of understanding the relationship between oral health and headache/migraine. Respondents with prior training were significantly more aware ($p < 0.001$) than those without prior training. Educating families ($p < 0.001$), frequency of patient encounters with headache ($p = 0.032$), coordination with healthcare providers ($p = 0.002$), and access to appropriate management resources ($p < 0.001$) were significant predictors of providers' awareness. **Conclusions:** Pediatric dental providers expressed strong interest in enhancing their knowledge of headache/migraine management, highlighting the value of integrating headache/migraine-related education into training programs and promoting greater interdisciplinary collaboration.

Keywords: headache and migraine management; healthcare collaboration; provider knowledge; chronic pain in children; orofacial pain; pediatric dentistry; pediatric headache disorders; oral–systemic health

1. Introduction

Migraine is one of the most common types of primary headache and ranks as the third-most prevalent disorder globally, posing a significant and disabling public health burden [1,2]. The International Classification of Headache Disorders 3rd edition (ICHD-3) categorizes migraine into two major subtypes, migraine with and without an aura, and defines diagnostic criteria based on frequency and duration, with attacks lasting 4–72 h and occurring on at least five separate occasions [3]. In pediatric populations, migraine is a leading causes of emergency department visits for recurrent headache, contributing to increased healthcare utilization, school absenteeism, and reduced quality of life [4]. However, diagnosis is often delayed and management complicated by limited provider awareness, distinct signs and symptoms compared to migraine manifestation in adults, and inadequate access to pediatric headache specialists [5]. In children and adolescents, diagnosis relies heavily on clinical history and symptom patterning, which may complicate recognition and prolong time to treatment initiation [6]. Although multidisciplinary approaches have shown promise, the literature remains scarce on management approaches in interdisciplinary or primary care settings [7].

Given that headaches (and particularly migraine) are a common comorbidity among patients with temporomandibular disorders (TMDs), and that both conditions share overlapping biological and psychosocial risk factors, there is a clear opportunity for greater interdisciplinary collaboration amongst pediatric oral healthcare providers [8,9]. Large-scale studies, including the OPPERA (Orofacial Pain: Prospective Evaluation and Risk Assessment) cohort, have shown that individuals with TMD are at significantly increased risk for developing migraine, likely due to shared mechanisms such as central sensitization, impaired pain modulation, and psychosocial stress [10–13]. These findings highlight the importance of early recognition and coordinated care strategies. Pediatric migraine may have lasting consequences that extend into adulthood, including physical, emotional and psychosocial effects [5,14]. Furthermore, symptom overlap between migraine and neurovascular orofacial pain (e.g., photophobia and phonophobia) can complicate diagnosis and lead to misattributed pain etiologies [5,15]. As frontline providers for pediatric orofacial pain complaints, pediatric dentists are uniquely positioned to support early recognition of migraine symptoms, especially when facial or jaw pain is the chief complaint, and to facilitate appropriate referral and care coordination. Although precise data are lacking, case series have described instances in which migraine was misdiagnosed as dental pain, resulting in unnecessary dental procedures such as extractions [16,17]. Pediatric dentists may support headache/migraine management by screening for hallmark symptoms during routine dental visits, including photophobia, phonophobia, nausea, or pain exacerbated by routine activities. When these features are present, providers can educate families about the potential link to headache disorders and refer the patient to a pediatrician or neurologist for further evaluation. Simple tools, such as symptom checklists or referral algorithms, could help integrate this process into routine care without significantly increasing visit time. While dentists receive training in the differential diagnosis of orofacial pain, formal instruction on the recognition and co-management of primary headache disorders, such as pediatric migraine, is often limited or absent in dental education. As a result, it remains unclear whether pediatric dentists feel their current knowledge is sufficient, or whether there is a need for continued education and refresher training, to recognize migraine-specific symptoms and contribute to interdisciplinary care for affected patients. While the Commission on Dental Accreditation (CODA) standards for pediatric dentistry (USA—2025) outlines essential competencies in the diagnosis and management of oral diseases and craniofacial development in pediatric populations, current curricula offer limited emphasis on primary headache disorders, including migraine, or on interdisciplinary care coordination for orofacial pain conditions that extend beyond the dentition [18].

Increased awareness among pediatric dentists could facilitate earlier referral to neurologists or pain specialists, ultimately improving patient outcomes and reducing the risk of misdiagnosis or unnecessary interventions. Additionally, given the emerging recognition of the relationship between oral parafunctional habits, such as clenching, bruxism, and TMD, and headache disorders, dental providers may be well-positioned to recommend behavioral interventions or deliver occlusal appliance therapies as adjuncts to comprehensive migraine management. However, the extent to which pediatric dental providers currently engage in headache/migraine-related care, feel equipped to do so, or express interest in expanding their role, remains largely unknown.

This study aimed to evaluate pediatric dentists' training, clinical experience, and perceived knowledge gaps related to pediatric headache/migraine, with the goal of identifying gaps that may inform future education and interdisciplinary care strategies. We hypothesized that pediatric dentists and residents would report limited formal training and low self-perceived awareness of the oral–systemic connections relevant to pediatric headache/migraine.

2. Materials and Methods

2.1. Study Design

This cross-sectional survey study was reviewed by the University of North Carolina Institutional Review Board (IRB) and deemed exempt (24-0459, 20 February 2025). An anonymous online questionnaire was distributed via Qualtrics to all members of the American Academy of Pediatric Dentistry (AAPD). Eligible participants needed to be completing or have already completed specialized training in pediatric dentistry at a U.S. CODA-accredited advanced dental education program. Electronic informed consent was obtained from respondents prior to participation. In accordance with local IRB regulations, participants were not obligated to respond to all survey items.

2.2. Survey Assessment Tool

The anonymous survey (Supplementary Materials) was co-developed by a pediatric dentist (C.M.S.), a pediatric dentistry resident (S.G.), and an orofacial pain specialist (L.S.), with expertise in pediatric dentistry (C.M.S., S.G.) and pediatric orofacial pain (L.S.). Survey content was also reviewed by external content experts to ensure relevance and appropriateness of questions, as well as readability and accessibility. The finalized survey was also reviewed by the Odum Institute for Research in Social Science at the University of North Carolina to evaluate survey structure, item clarity, and formatting. While content review was conducted by subject matter experts, the instrument has not yet undergone formal psychometric validation. While the term "headache/migraine" does not appear as such in the International Classification of Headache Disorders (ICHD-3), this phrasing has been used to be inclusive of different forms of headache and migraine. This wording enables a more relevant clinical application for the population of our study. The final survey consisted of 28 items across 5 sections. Responses to all sections were optional. Section 1 assessed respondents' professional background, years of experience, additional training on pediatric headaches/migraine, location of work and primary practice setting. Section 2 evaluated general understanding and provider's knowledge into an oral health and headache/migraine link, as well as experience in educating families in practice. Section 3 involved questions on patient identification and practice interventions, inquiring on frequency of identified patients as well as frequency of counseling and working with an interdisciplinary pediatric headache team. Section 4 included questions on pediatric dentists' opinion on their role in headache/migraine management as well as future focused questions on implementation into practice. The final section of this survey assessed sociodemographic characteristics. Opportunities to elaborate on close-ended responses were provided throughout the process via optional open text boxes.

2.3. Data Analysis

Descriptive statistics were used to summarize respondents' demographic, professional characteristics, and study variables. Differences in providers' general understanding of the link between oral conditions and headache/migraine were examined across years of professional experience using a one-way analysis of variance (ANOVA), with Bonferroni as post hoc test for comparison.

Next, subgroup analyses were computed. Independent *t*-tests compared respondents with and without prior dedicated training in headache/migraine prevention, access to adequate resources, and engagement in related behaviors (e.g., educating patients' families) in terms of their general understanding. Chi-square tests were used to investigate whether frequency of encountering patients reporting headaches/migraine differed based on years of professional experience, family education behaviors, opportunities for interprofessional coordination, and approaches to managing pediatric headache/migraine. Effect sizes were reported using Cohen's *d* for *t*-tests, Cramer's V for chi-square tests, and eta-squared (η^2) for ANOVAs. According to conventional thresholds, an effect size of 0.2 is considered small, 0.5 medium, and 0.8 large [19].

Finally, a multiple linear regression model was conducted to identify predictors of providers' awareness of the link between oral conditions and pediatric headache/migraine.

All the analyses were conducted with SPSS (IBM SPSS Statistics Macintosh, Version 29.00, IBM Corp., Armonk, NY, USA), setting α at <0.05.

3. Results

3.1. Participants

Out of 367 total responses, 5 (1.4%) derived from participants who did not complete or were not currently completing a specialized training in pediatric dentistry, while 47 (12.8%) were submitted without any data. Thus, these entries were excluded from the final analysis, leaving a total of 315 participants (Figure 1). Based on 315 completed surveys out of approximately 6500 reachable AAPD members, the response rate was 4.8%.

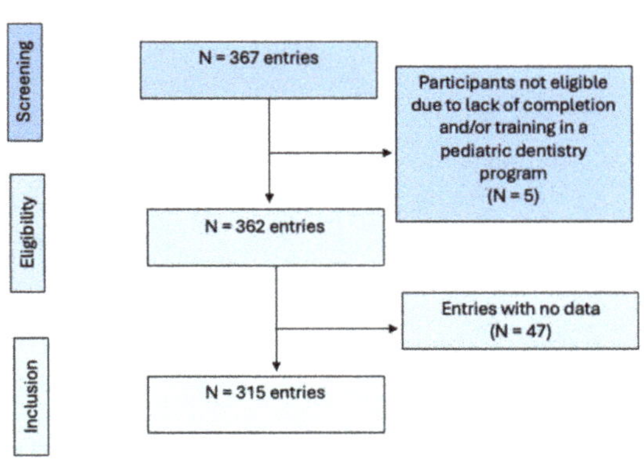

Figure 1. Flowchart of study participants.

Most of the respondents (81.6%) were practicing pediatric dentists primarily working in private practice (66.0%) and academia (21.3%), while 15.9% of the responses derived from pediatric dental residents. Most of the participants indicated working in suburban (53.0%) and urban areas (36.5%). Almost half of the respondents (46.3%) had over 20 years of experience. Demographic characteristics of the total sample are presented in Table 1.

Table 1. Demographic characteristics of participants.

Variables	Answer Options	Total (N = 315)
Age	25–29 years old	33 (10.5%)
	30–39 years old	66 (21.0%)
	40–49 years old	59 (18.7%)
	50–59 years old	65 (20.6%)
	60 or older	72 (22.9%)
	Prefer not to answer	2 (0.6%)
	Missing	18 (5.7%)
Sex	Male	133 (42.2%)
	Female	162 (51.4%)
	Prefer not to answer	2 (0.6%)
	Missing	18 (5.7%)
Ethnicity	Hispanic or Latinx	17 (5.4%)
	Not Hispanic or Latinx	255 (81.0%)
	Prefer not to answer	25 (7.9%)
	Missing	18 (5.7%)
Race	White	219 (69.5%)
	Black or African American	16 (5.1%)
	Asian	39 (12.4%)
	Other	6 (1.9%)
	Prefer not to answer	17 (5.4%)
	Missing	18 (5.7%)
Professional role	Retired pediatric dentist	8 (2.5%)
	Practicing pediatric dentist	257 (81.6%)
	Pediatric dental resident	50 (15.9%)
Practice setting	Private practice	208 (66.0%)
	Academia	67 (21.3%)
	Private practice and academia	27 (8.6%)
	Community/public health clinic	11 (3.5%)
	Other	2 (0.6%)
Type of location	Urban	115 (36.5%)
	Suburban	167 (53.0%)
	Rural	33 (10.5%)
Region of practice	Northeast	90 (28.6%)
	Midwest	58 (18.4%)
	West	60 (19.0%)
	Southeast	74 (23.5%)
	Southwest	33 (10.5%)
Years of experience	0–5 years	83 (26.3%)
	6–10 years	34 (10.8%)
	11–15 years	30 (9.5%)
	16–20 years	22 (7.0%)
	Over 20 years	146 (46.3%)

Values are presented as frequencies and percentages.

3.2. Providers' General Understanding

On average, respondents reported a self-perceived awareness score of 2.7 ± 1.3 (on a 0–5 numerical rating scale) regarding the potential contribution of oral conditions to headache/migraine in pediatric patients. The most frequently identified contributing factors were clenching (73.7%), bruxism (72.4%), and TMD (65.7%), among others (Figure 2A). A majority of respondents (85.2%) estimated that less than 50% of their pediatric patients exhibited parafunctional habits such as teeth grinding or clenching (Figure 2B).

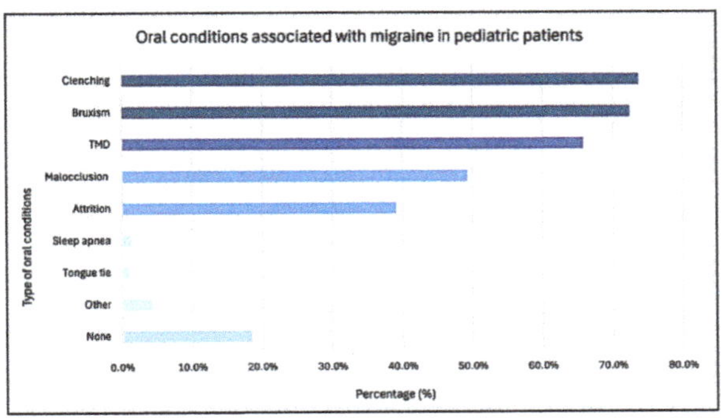

(A)

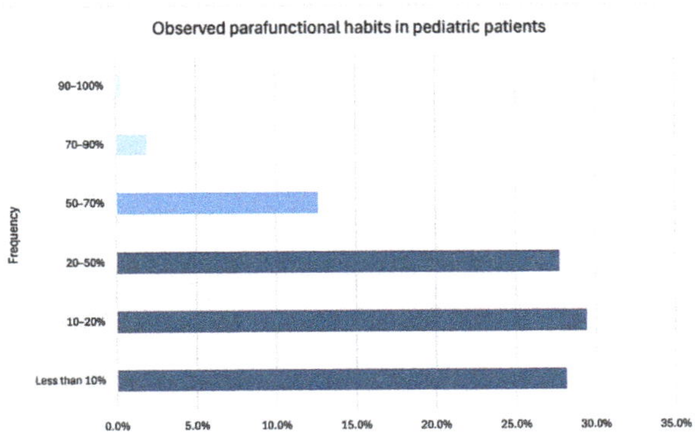

(B)

Figure 2. Type of oral conditions perceived to be associated with headache/migraine in pediatric patients (**A**), frequency of observed parafunctional habits (**B**).

Pediatric dentists with over 20 years of experience reported significantly higher awareness of this connection (4.5 ± 0.9) compared to those with 0–5 years (3.3 ± 1.7, $p = 0.015$), 6–10 years (2.9 ± 1.8, $p < 0.001$), and 11–15 years of experience (3.3 ± 1.8, $p = 0.007$, Figure 3A). These differences in awareness occurred despite no significant differences in reported training on the role of pediatric dentists in migraine prevention or management during their education ($X^2(4) = 1.176$, $p = 0.882$).

A large majority (95.2%) indicated that their formal educational background did not include training on the role of pediatric dentists in headache/migraine prevention or management. Only 34.2% felt they were equipped with resources to address the potential oral health–headache/migraine connection. Respondents who reported being equipped with such resources demonstrated significantly higher awareness of their link compared to those who were not (3.4 ± 1.3 vs. 2.4 ± 1.1, $p < 0.001$, Cohen's $d = 0.91$). Similarly, only 24.4% reported educating families on the relationship between oral conditions and headache/migraine in their pediatric patients. Those who had received headache/migraine-related training (N = 15) and those who reported educating families on the oral condition–headache/migraine connection (N = 77) also demonstrated significantly higher awareness compared to those who did not receive any training (3.3 ± 1.1 vs. 2.7 ± 1.3, $p = 0.049$, Cohen's $d = 0.52$, Figure 3B) and those who did not educate the families on such a link (3.6 ± 1.2 vs. 2.4 ± 1.1, $p < 0.001$, Cohen's $d = 0.99$, Figure 3C).

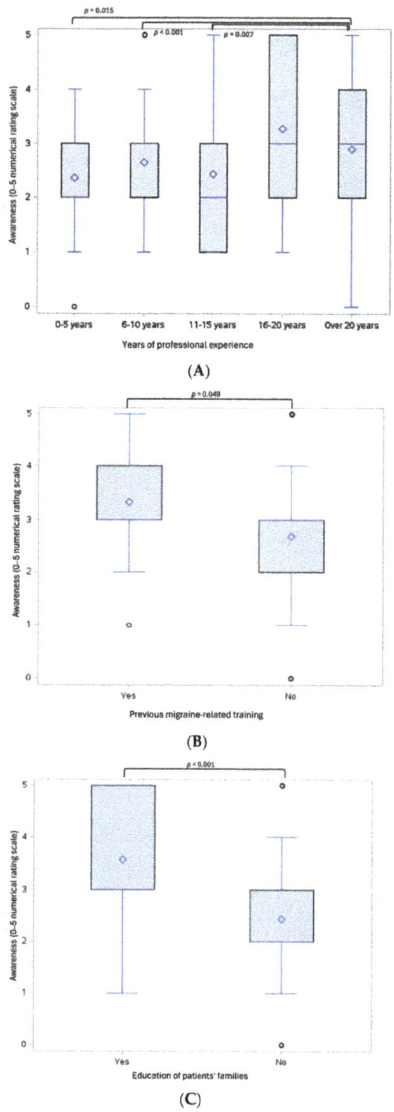

Figure 3. Box plots illustrating statistically significant differences in pediatric dentists' awareness of the link between oral conditions and pediatric headache/migraine (measured on a 5-point Likert scale), based on years of professional experience (**A**), previous headache/migraine-related training (**B**), and behaviors related to educating patients' families (**C**). ◇ represents the mean; ○ represents outliers, which fall outside 1.5 times the interquartile range (IRQ) from the lower or upper quartiles.

A multiple regression was performed to predict providers' awareness of the oral conditions-headache/migraine connection based on previous migraine-related training, years of professional experience, interprofessional collaboration, access to management resources, family education behaviors, and frequency of patient encounters involving headaches. The model significantly predicted providers' awareness ($F(6, 303) = 19.873$, $p < 0.001$, $R^2 = 0.268$). Specifically, educating families ($p < 0.001$), frequency of patient encounters with headache ($p = 0.032$), coordination with other healthcare providers ($p = 0.002$), and access to appropriate management resources ($p < 0.001$) were statistically significant predictors.

3.3. Patient Identification and Practice Interventions

Over two-thirds of respondents (71.0%) indicated that their pediatric patients rarely complain about headaches during their consultation or rarely seek advice from their pediatric dentist regarding headaches, without any differences based on type of primary practice setting ($X^2(12) = 13.616$, $p = 0.326$, Cramer's V = 0.12). However, providers with 20 or more years of experience were significantly more likely to encounter pediatric patients who complained about headaches either frequently (2.8%) or occasionally (19.3%) compared to their less experienced counterparts ($X^2(12) = 22.815$, $p = 0.029$, Cramer's V = 0.27). Respondents who reported educating families on the connection between oral conditions and headache/migraine were also more likely to have patients complaining either frequently (5.2% vs. 0.0%) or occasionally (24.7% vs. 10.3%) compared to those who did not provide such education to their patients ($X^2(3) = 25.521$, $p < 0.001$, Cramer's V = 0.29). Those providers also reported significantly more patients who actively sought advice about headaches during consultations, either frequently (5.2% vs. 0.4%) or occasionally (20.8% vs. 3.9%, $X^2(3) = 47.088$, $p < 0.001$, Cramer's V = 0.39). Moreover, providers who encountered pediatric patients complaining of headache were more likely to coordinate care with other healthcare professionals, such as pediatricians, neurologists, and orofacial pain specialists ($X^2(3) = 29.111$, $p < 0.001$, Cramer's V = 0.31). They were also more likely to report being equipped with resources to address the oral health–headache/migraine connection ($X^2(3) = 10.339$, $p = 0.016$, Cramer's V = 0.18) and to actively collaborate in managing pediatric migraine ($X^2(6) = 25.833$, $p < 0.001$, Cramer's V = 0.30). Similarly, respondents whose patients frequently (3.5% vs. 0.0%) or occasionally (16.0% vs. 1.2%) sought advice about headache were more likely to coordinate interprofessional care ($X^2(3) = 59.774$, $p < 0.001$) and to be involved in headache/migraine management ($X^2(6) = 49.873$, $p < 0.001$, Cramer's V = 0.41).

The most common recommended approaches for headache/migraine management included nighttime occlusal appliances (50.8%), followed by referral to medical (47.0%) and dental (42.5%) specialists, orthodontic therapies (43.8%), and stress management strategies (35.9%, Figure 4).

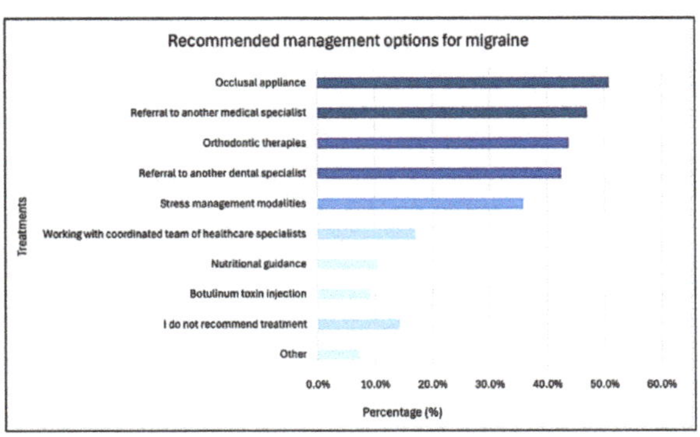

Figure 4. Recommended treatment management for migraine in pediatric dental patients.

3.4. Provider Opinion and Future Focus

As high as 78.1% agreed—either somewhat (45.2%) or strongly (32.9%)—that it is important for pediatric dentists to understand the oral health–headache/migraine relationship.

Additionally, 85.5% of respondents endorsed the need for increased interdisciplinary collaboration in the management of pediatric headache/migraine. Similarly, 83.2% expressed the need for further training and research in this area. Preferred modalities included continuing education courses (71.7%), integration into pediatric dental residency curricula (56.5%), and more lectures at the AAPD annual session, among others (Figure 5).

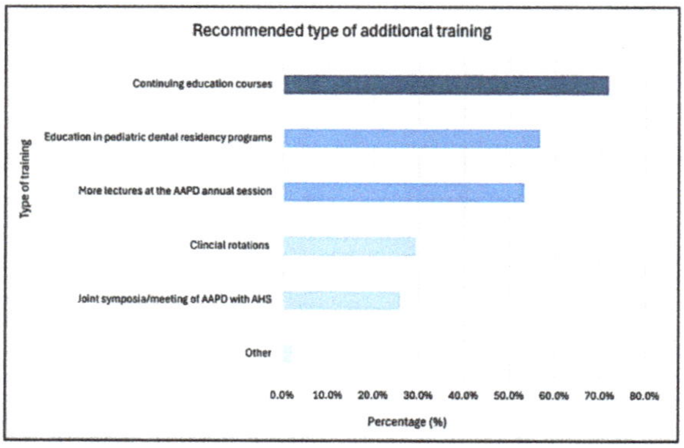

Figure 5. Recommended resources of additional training for pediatric headache/migraine management. AAPD: American Academy of Pediatric Dentistry; AHS: American Headache Society.

The most frequently reported barriers to implementing headache/migraine management into practice were lack of training of formal training or education on the topic (73.7%), limited collaboration with other healthcare providers (36.5%), challenges in distinguishing between dental pain and headache/migraine symptoms (30.8%), and time constraints (28.9%). Only 2.1% of respondents believed that pediatric dentists should not be involved in headache/migraine management in their pediatric patients (Figure 6).

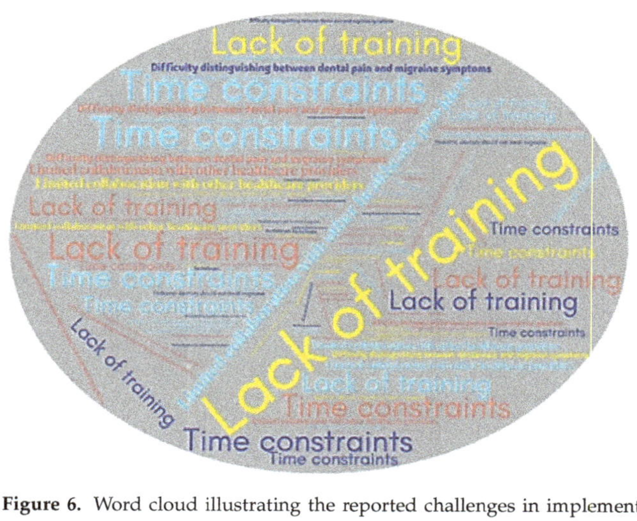

Figure 6. Word cloud illustrating the reported challenges in implementing headache/migraine management into pediatric dentistry practice. Larger size and more frequently repeated items reflect challenges more commonly mentioned by respondents.

4. Discussion

Despite headaches and, specifically migraine, having reciprocal linkages with clinical findings in the pediatric dental setting, this topic remains underemphasized in current training programs and continuing education. The findings of this survey support our initial hypothesis that pediatric dentists and residents report limited formal training and low self-perceived awareness of the oral–systemic connections relevant to pediatric headache/migraine. Respondents' mean awareness score of 2.7 ± 1.3 (on a 0–5 numerical rating scale) regarding the contribution of oral conditions to headache/migraine highlights an area of opportunity for further education in this area. While the study did not evaluate clinical outcomes, the reported lack of formal training and limited awareness among providers suggest opportunities for ongoing education to strengthen interdisciplinary care for pediatric patients experiencing headache/migraine. Although the AAPD acknowledges primary headaches as common in childhood and adolescence and describes migraine among potential sources of orofacial pain, current guidelines do not include diagnostic criteria for screening and recognition or co-management strategies for migraine. It is important to note that pediatric dentists are not expected to diagnose migraine, but rather to recognize when a child's symptoms may be consistent with migraine or other primary headache disorders, and to facilitate appropriate referral to a medical provider for diagnosis and management. However, such content is largely absent from pediatric dental curricula and training programs [18,20,21].

It is possible that clinical experience and time in the field contribute to greater awareness, as pediatric dentists with over 20 years of experience reported a significantly higher awareness of a connection between oral health and headache/migraine. This is notable, as these differences in awareness occurred despite no reported differences in training on the role of pediatric dentists in headache/migraine prevention or management during their education. In fact, only 34.2% of respondents felt they were equipped with the resources to address the potential oral health–headache/migraine connection. Additionally, the most frequently identified contributing factors included clenching, bruxism, and TMD. It is also important to note that while the survey focused on migraine, some reported associations, such as those involving parafunctional habits or TMD, may reflect broader provider beliefs about headache etiology rather than migraine specifically. While some literature supports associations between these factors and pediatric headache, research on this link remains limited and methodologically challenging to study in pediatric populations [22]. Effective pediatric care extends beyond treating oral health in isolation but understanding the child in a broader context of their emotional, psychosocial, and overall well-being.

The need for interdisciplinary care and education resources in this realm extends beyond dentistry. The American Headache Society, for example, has developed the "First Contact-Headache in Primary Care" program to provide healthcare providers with the tools to improve headache and migraine care access [23]. The importance of working with interdisciplinary teams cannot be overstated as the ability to coordinate with and refer to other healthcare professionals, such as pediatricians, neurologists, orofacial pain specialists, may be essential for patients debilitated by migraine. Notably, 85.5% of respondents endorsed the need for enhanced interdisciplinary collaboration in pediatric headache/migraine management. Multifaceted, team-based approaches have shown effectiveness in addressing this condition by targeting its intricate etiologies [7].

While headache/migraine management may not be a component of formal education within pediatric dentistry, the findings of this study highlight a call to action to proactively educate early-career providers in this field. This need is further supported by the finding that respondents who felt equipped with educational resources and understanding demonstrated significantly greater awareness of the potential connection between oral health conditions with migraine in pediatric populations. Among respondents, the greatest barrier to implementing headache/migraine management into practice was lack of formal training or education on the topic. Similar gaps in training have also been reported internationally. For instance, a survey of Brazilian orthodontists found that although many providers encountered patients with migraine symptoms, most felt unprepared to diagnose or manage them due to a lack of formal education in headache-related care [24]. These findings highlight a broader, global need to integrate content on headache disorders and interdisciplinary pain management into dental education and continuing professional development.

The distinction in pathophysiological mechanisms between adult and pediatric migraine, largely due to continuous neural development in children, situates pediatric dentists in a unique role for prompt recognition of orofacial pain symptoms, facilitating both proactive clinical response and timely referrals [25]. Because migraine research and pharmacological interventions have traditionally focused on adult populations, directly extrapolating findings to pediatric populations is often unreliable, and unaddressed migraine symptoms in childhood may carry significant long-term consequences. Non-pharmacological treatments, such as cognitive behavior therapy, have demonstrated efficacy in reducing chronic migraine episodes in children and are often most effective when integrated with pharmacologic approaches [26]. Given that adults with migraines frequently experience comorbid anxiety and depression, early identification and management of pediatric somatic symptoms is critical to mitigating long-term psychological and functional impact [26,27]. For pediatric dental providers, awareness of migraine signs and symptoms is especially important due to their overlap with TMD-related pain and associated functional limitations, as well as the risk of psychological distress that may exacerbate orofacial pain conditions over time [14,28,29].

Open dialogue between providers and families is essential, yet if pediatric dental providers are unaware of the potential connection between oral conditions and headache/migraine, key symptoms may go unrecognized or unreported during visits. In fact, respondents who reported educating families on the connection between oral conditions and headache/migraine were also more likely to have patients complaining either frequently (5.2% vs. 0.0%) or occasionally (24.7% vs. 10.3%) compared to those who did not provide such education. These findings suggest that provider awareness directly influences patient disclosures, reinforcing that education begins with a strong knowledge base and the ability to inquire effectively about relevant symptoms and medical history. When equipped with this knowledge, providers are better positioned to refer, educate, and support families appropriately.

Given the frequency of biannual preventive visits, and potentially more for restorative or behavioral concerns, pediatric dentists often maintain more consistent clinical contact with children than many other providers. With only 2.1% of respondents believing that pediatric dentists should not be involved in headache/migraine management, it is evident that both perceived value and professional interest are high. However, greater emphasis on headache/migraine recognition and referral strategies within pediatric dental training and continuing education may be needed to fully integrate this role into routine practice.

Findings from this study illustrate a knowledge gap not only across different generations of pediatric dentists and residents, but also within educational content and interdisciplinary care models. Similar studies piloting interprofessional healthcare approaches in pediatric medicine and dentistry have shown promise in improving referral pathways and care coordination [30]. Future research could explore the development and evaluation of online training modules or continuing education programs, incorporating feedback from pediatric dentists and residents on content retention and clinical applicability. Additionally, integrating dentistry into headache teams or pediatric headache/migraine clinics may provide a practical framework to foster interdisciplinary collaboration.

The results described above should be interpreted in light of the study's limitations. The response rate was modest (~4.8%), which limits generalizability and raises the potential for non-response bias. It is likely that individuals with greater interest in headache/migraine or orofacial pain were more inclined to participate. However, similar response rates have been reported in prior studies surveying pediatric dental providers, including those evaluating pain management practices and TMD screening behaviors, suggesting that the rate observed here is consistent with research in this field [31,32]. A second limitation is sampling bias, as responses were collected only from AAPD members and may not be representative of the broader pediatric dental community. Additionally, the voluntary nature of survey participation introduces the potential for non-response bias, whereby individuals with limited interest or knowledge of the topic may have been less likely to respond, thus potentially skewing findings toward participants with stronger engagement or opinions. Finally, the small number of respondents with formal headache/migraine-related training limits subgroup comparisons and highlights the need for additional research with larger and more diverse samples. While our study did not evaluate whether insufficient training leads to diagnostic errors or treatment delays, the findings highlight a widespread interest in additional guidance related to headache/migraine, indicating that pediatric dental providers themselves perceive this as a relevant clinical and educational need

5. Conclusions

The findings of this study revealed that the vast majority of respondents had not received formal education related to pediatric headache/migraine and reported low self-perceived awareness of the link between oral health and headache/migraine symptoms. Despite this, most participants believed that pediatric dentists should understand this relationship and expressed strong interest in additional training opportunities and interdisciplinary collaboration. Providers who had received headache/migraine-related training, educated families on the topic, or coordinated care with other professionals were significantly more aware of migraine–oral health connections. These findings highlight a need to improve educational content related to pediatric headache/migraine within dental curricula and continuing education programs, with an emphasis on early recognition, family communication, and referral pathways. Improved access to targeted education in this area may enhance care coordination, reduce misdiagnosis or inappropriate management, and ultimately support more comprehensive, patient-centered care, while also strengthening collaboration across pediatric healthcare teams.

Supplementary Materials: The following supporting information can be downloaded at https://www.mdpi.com/article/10.3390/children12080968/s1, Survey used in the current study.

Author Contributions: Conceptualization, C.M.S., S.G. and L.S.; Methodology, C.M.S. and S.G.; Formal Analysis, L.S.; Investigation, C.M.S. and S.G.; Resources, C.M.S. and S.G.; Data Curation, S.G.; Writing—Original Draft Preparation, C.M.S. and S.G.; Writing—Review and Editing, L.S.; Project Administration, C.M.S. All authors have read and agreed to the published version of the manuscript.

Funding: This research received no external funding.

Institutional Review Board Statement: The study (24-0459) was reviewed by the Office of Human Research Ethics and was determined to be exempt from further review according to the regulatory category cited above under 45 CFR 46.104, 20 February 2025.

Informed Consent Statement: At the outset of the survey, participants encountered a consent statement clearly stating their voluntary agreement to participate in the survey. To proceed with the survey, participants must have explicitly agreed to the consent statement by clicking on a designated "I agree" button.

Data Availability Statement: The original contributions presented in the study are included in the article/Supplementary Materials; further inquiries can be directed to the corresponding author.

Conflicts of Interest: The authors declare no conflicts of interest.

Abbreviations

The following abbreviations are used in this manuscript:

CODA	Commission on Dental Accreditation
ICHD	International Classification of Headache Disorders
TMD	Temporomandibular Disorder
AHS	American Headache Society
AAPD	American Academy of Pediatric Dentistry
CBT	Cognitive Behavioral Therapy

References

1. Ahmed, F. Headache Disorders: Differentiating and Managing the Common Subtypes. *Br. J. Pain* **2012**, *6*, 124–132. [CrossRef] [PubMed]
2. Stovner, L.; Hagen, K.; Jensen, R.; Katsarava, Z.; Lipton, R.; Scher, A.; Steiner, T.; Zwart, J.-A. The Global Burden of Headache: A Documentation of Headache Prevalence and Disability Worldwide. *Cephalalgia* **2007**, *27*, 193–210. [CrossRef] [PubMed]
3. Gobel, H. Classification. Available online: https://ichd-3.org/classification-outline/ (accessed on 28 May 2025).
4. O'Brien, H.L.; Kabbouche, M.A.; Kacperski, J.; Hershey, A.D. Treatment of Pediatric Migraine. *Curr. Treat. Options Neurol.* **2015**, *17*, 1. [CrossRef]
5. Khan, A.; Liu, S.; Tao, F. Current Trends in Pediatric Migraine: Clinical Insights and Therapeutic Strategies. *Brain Sci.* **2025**, *15*, 280. [CrossRef]
6. Dooley, J. The Evaluation and Management of Paediatric Headaches. *Paediatr. Child Health* **2009**, *14*, 24–30. [CrossRef]
7. Esparham, A.; Herbert, A.; Pierzchalski, E.; Tran, C.; Dilts, J.; Boorigie, M.; Wingert, T.; Connelly, M.; Bickel, J. Pediatric Headache Clinic Model: Implementation of Integrative Therapies in Practice. *Children* **2018**, *5*, 74. [CrossRef]
8. Wagner, B.D.A.; Moreira Filho, P.F. Painful Temporomandibular Disorder, Sleep Bruxism, Anxiety Symptoms and Subjective Sleep Quality among Military Firefighters with Frequent Episodic Tension-Type Headache. A Controlled Study. *Arq. Neuropsiquiatr.* **2018**, *76*, 387–392. [CrossRef]
9. Silva Júnior, A.A.D.; Brandão, K.V.; Faleiros, B.E.; Tavares, R.M.; Lara, R.P.; Januzzi, E.; Carvalho, A.B.D.; Carvalho, E.M.D.D.; Gomes, J.B.L.; Leite, F.M.G.; et al. Temporo-Mandibular Disorders Are an Important Comorbidity of Migraine and May Be Clinically Difficult to Distinguish Them from Tension-Type Headache. *Arq. Neuropsiquiatr.* **2014**, *72*, 99–103. [CrossRef]
10. Gonçalves, D.A.G.; Camparis, C.M.; Speciali, J.G.; Franco, A.L.; Castanharo, S.M.; Bigal, M.E. Temporomandibular Disorders Are Differentially Associated with Headache Diagnoses: A Controlled Study. *Clin. J. Pain* **2011**, *27*, 611–615. [CrossRef]
11. Tchivileva, I.E.; Ohrbach, R.; Fillingim, R.B.; Greenspan, J.D.; Maixner, W.; Slade, G.D. Temporal Change in Headache and Its Contribution to the Risk of Developing First-Onset Temporomandibular Disorder in the Orofacial Pain: Prospective Evaluation and Risk Assessment (OPPERA) Study. *Pain* **2017**, *158*, 120–129. [CrossRef]
12. Goncalves, D.A.G.; Camparis, C.M.; Speciali, J.G.; Castanharo, S.M.; Ujikawa, L.T.; Lipton, R.B.; Bigal, M.E. Treatment of Comorbid Migraine and Temporomandibular Disorders: A Factorial, Double-Blind, Randomized, Placebo-Controlled Study. *J. Orofac. Pain.* **2013**, *27*, 325–335. [CrossRef]
13. Gonçalves, D.A.G.; Bigal, M.E.; Jales, L.C.F.; Camparis, C.M.; Speciali, J.G. Headache and Symptoms of Temporomandibular Disorder: An Epidemiological Study. *Headache J. Head Face Pain* **2010**, *50*, 231–241. [CrossRef]
14. Rizvi, B.A.; Kuziek, J.; Cho, L.Y.; Ronksley, P.E.; Noel, M.N.; Orr, S.L. Anxiety and Depressive Symptoms and Migraine-related Outcomes in Children and Adolescents. *Headache J. Head Face Pain* **2024**, *64*, 342–351. [CrossRef]
15. Benoliel, R.; May, A. Orofacial Migraine—A Narrative Review. *J. Clin. Med.* **2024**, *13*, 5745. [CrossRef]
16. Peñarrocha, M.; Bandrés, A.; Peñarrocha, M.; Bagán, J.V. Lower-Half Facial Migraine: A Report of 11 Cases. *J. Oral Maxillofac. Surg. Off. J. Am. Assoc. Oral Maxillofac. Surg.* **2004**, *62*, 1453–1456. [CrossRef]

17. Lambru, G.; Elias, L.-A.; Yakkaphan, P.; Renton, T. Migraine Presenting as Isolated Facial Pain: A Prospective Clinical Analysis of 58 Cases. *Cephalalgia* **2020**, *40*, 1250–1254. [CrossRef] [PubMed]
18. Commission on Dental Accreditation. *Accreditation Standards for Advanced Dental Education Programs in Pediatric Dentistry*; American Dental Association: Chicago, IL, USA, 2025.
19. Cohen, J. *Statistical Power Analysis for the Behavioral Sciences*, 2nd ed.; reprint; Psychology Press: New York, NY, USA, 2009; ISBN 978-0-8058-0283-2.
20. American Academy of Pediatric Dentistry. Pain Management in Infants, Children, Adolescents, and Individuals with Special Health Care Needs. In *The Reference Manual of Pediatric Dentistry*; American Academy of Pediatric Dentistry: Chicago, IL, USA, 2024; pp. 435–443.
21. American Academy of Pediatric Dentistry. Temporomandibular Disorders in Children and Adolescents, Including Those with Special Health Care Needs. In *The Reference Manual of Pediatric Dentistry*; American Academy of Pediatric Dentistry: Chicago, IL, USA, 2024; pp. 494–504.
22. Nascimento, M.C.P.D.; Melo, T.F.A.O.; da Luz Neto, R.G.; Silveira, M.A.C.D.; Vieira, S.C.M.; Heimer, M.V. Sleep Bruxism, Awake Bruxism and Headache in Children and Adolescents: A Scoping Review. *J. Oral Facial Pain Headache* **2024**, *38*, 1–10. [CrossRef] [PubMed]
23. Minen, M.T.; Malhotra, N.A.; Waire, E.K.; Swiderski, H.Z.; Riggins, N.Y.; Sprouse-Blum, A.S. The American Headache Society First Contact—Headache in Primary Care Program: Current Metrics, Knowledge Assessments, and Direction for Future Initiatives. *Headache J. Head Face Pain* **2025**, *65*, 280–290. [CrossRef] [PubMed]
24. Junior, R.L.M.; de Carvalho Kerber, F.; Stuginski-Barbosa, J. Attitudes of a Group of Brazilian Orthodontists towards the Diagnosis and Management of Primary Headache (Migraine): An Electronic-Based Survey. *J. Appl. Oral Sci. Rev. FOB* **2011**, *19*, 674–678. [CrossRef]
25. Førland-Schill, A.; Berring-Uldum, A.; Debes, N.M. Migraine Pathophysiology in Children and Adolescents: A Review of the Literature. *J. Child Neurol.* **2022**, *37*, 642–651. [CrossRef]
26. Kroner, J.W.; Hershey, A.D.; Kashikar-Zuck, S.M.; LeCates, S.L.; Allen, J.R.; Slater, S.K.; Zafar, M.; Kabbouche, M.A.; O'Brien, H.L.; Shenk, C.E.; et al. Cognitive Behavioral Therapy plus Amitriptyline for Children and Adolescents with Chronic Migraine Reduces Headache Days to $\leq$4 Per Month. *Headache J. Head Face Pain* **2016**, *56*, 711–716. [CrossRef] [PubMed]
27. Ziółkiewicz, A.; Jartych, A.; Iwanicka, K.; Chawrylak, K.; Zegardło, W.; Szukała, K.; Chrościńska-Krawczyk, M. Migraines in Childhood as a Cause of Headache in Adulthood—How to Prevent It? A Literature Review. *J. Pre-Clin. Clin. Res.* **2024**, *1*, 74–82. [CrossRef]
28. Nilsson, I.-M.; List, T.; Drangsholt, M. Headache and Co-Morbid Pains Associated with TMD Pain in Adolescents. *J. Dent. Res.* **2013**, *92*, 802–807. [CrossRef] [PubMed]
29. Branco, L.P.; Santis, T.O.; Alfaya, T.A.; Godoy, C.H.L.; Fragoso, Y.D.; Bussadori, S.K. Association between Headache and Temporomandibular Joint Disorders in Children and Adolescents. *J. Oral Sci.* **2013**, *55*, 39–43. [CrossRef] [PubMed]
30. Niranjan, R.; Kim, J.; Lin, B.; Lewis, S.; Patel, P.; Le, T.; Alkon, A.; Chen, J.-L. Pediatric Dental Education Improves Interprofessional Healthcare Students' Clinical Competence in Children's Oral Health Assessment. *Dent. J.* **2019**, *7*, 106. [CrossRef]
31. Pielech, M.; Sawicki, C.M. Provider Perspectives on Pain Management Practices and Needs in Pediatric Dentistry. *J. Am. Dent. Assoc. 1939* **2023**, *154*, 1067–1076. [CrossRef]
32. Sawicki, C.M.; Sangalli, L. Pediatric Dentists' Practice Patterns in the Screening, Diagnosis, and Management of Temporomandibular Disorders. *Children* **2024**, *11*, 1168. [CrossRef]

children

MDPI

Article

How Can Specialist Advice Influence the Neuroimaging Practice for Childhood Headache in Emergency Department?

Alberto M. Cappellari [1,*], Gaia Bruschi [2], Gisella B. Beretta [2], Maria T. Molisso [1] and Giuseppe Bertolozzi [3]

1 Department of Neuroscience and Mental Health, Fondazione IRCCS Ca' Granda Ospedale Maggiore Policlinico, 20122 Milan, Italy; maria.molisso@policlinico.mi.it
2 Postgraduate School of Paediatrics, Università degli Studi di Milano, 20122 Milan, Italy; gaia.bruschi@unimi.it (G.B.); gisella.beretta@unimi.it (G.B.B.)
3 Pediatric Emergency Department, Fondazione IRCCS Ca' Granda Ospedale Maggiore Policlinico, 20122 Milan, Italy; giuseppe.bertolozzi@policlinico.mi.it
* Correspondence: alberto.cappellari@policlinico.mi.it; Tel.: +3902-5503-2406

Abstract: Differentiating between primary and secondary headaches can be challenging, especially in the emergency department (ED). Since symptoms alone are inadequate criteria for distinguishing between primary and secondary headaches, many children with headaches undergo neuroimaging investigations, such as brain CT and MRI. In various studies, the frequency of neuroimaging utilization is influenced by several factors, including teaching status, ownership, metropolitan area, insurance status, and ethnicity of patients. However, only a few studies have considered the role of specialist consultations in ordering neuroimaging studies on childhood headaches. We report the contributions of different specialists to the evaluation of children with headaches admitted to the ED and their influence on neuroimaging decisions. We retrospectively reviewed the medical reports of paediatric patients who presented with headaches to the paediatric ED of the Ospedale Maggiore Policlinico of Milano between January 2017 and January 2022. Overall, 890 children with headaches were evaluated (mean age: 10.0 years; range: 1 to 17 years). All patients were examined by the ED paediatricians, while specialist consultations were required for 261 patients, including 240 neurological (92.0%), 46 ophthalmological (17.6%), and 20 otorhinolaryngological (7.7%) consultations. Overall, 173 neuroimaging examinations were required, of which 51.4 and 48.6% were ordered by paediatricians and neurologists, respectively. In particular, paediatricians required 61.4% of brain CT scans, and neurologists required 92.0% of brain MRI scans. In conclusion, paediatricians were responsible for the management of most children with headaches admitted to the ED, while specialist consultations were required only in about a third of the cases. Although there was no significant difference in the number of neuroimaging studies ordered by specialists, brain CT scans were most often used by paediatricians, and MRI scans by neurologists.

Keywords: brain CT; brain MRI; neuroimaging; paediatrician; emergency department

1. Introduction

Headache is a common symptom in children and adolescents. The prevalence of headaches ranges from 5.9 to 37.7% in children and increases to 40–50% in school-age children and 80% in adolescents [1]. Severe headaches are known to cause anxiety in both children and parents and are a common reason of visits to the paediatric emergency department (ED) [2]. Many children are admitted to the emergency department with headaches every year, accounting for approximately 1% of ED visits [3]. The primary aim of clinicians in the paediatric ED is to recognize serious life-threatening conditions requiring immediate medical care among the wide spectrum of headache diagnoses. In less severe headache types, another objective is to perform appropriate evaluations and investigations to avoid unnecessary hospitalizations [2].

Primary headaches are syndromes in which headache is not a disease process, whereas secondary headaches are disorders in which headache represents a symptom of an underlying pathological process [4]. Primary headaches in children include migraine, migraine variants, tension-type headaches, and trigeminal autonomic cephalalgias [5]. Clinical manifestations of childhood primary headaches differ from those of adults, mainly due to differences in the degree of brain maturation, including myelination, plasticity, and synaptic reorganization [5,6]. Clinical features, risk factors, and aetiologies have a strong biopsychosocial basis in childhood, distinguishing primary headache disorders in children from those in adults [6]. Therefore, diagnosing primary headaches in young children can be challenging [7]. Secondary headache disorders in children differ from those in adults [6]. Clinicians should be aware of the specific features of secondary headache disorders in children to provide effective diagnosis and management [6].

Many studies in paediatric emergency settings have reported that viral infections, particularly respiratory tract infections (pharyngitis, tonsillitis, pneumonia, sinusitis, otitis, and adenoiditis) or minor head trauma, are the most common causes of secondary headaches [2,8,9].

Although most children suffer from primary headaches or headaches caused by self-limiting diseases, a small percentage have intracranial disorders [1]. It is necessary to detect serious underlying causes, such as brain tumors, viral and bacterial meningitis, and idiopathic intracranial hypertension [2]. Many clinical features, including preschool age, recent onset of headaches, occipital location, and neurological signs, could be useful for detecting secondary headaches due to intracranial disorders [2]. To identify serious etiologies of headaches in children and avoid unnecessary testing, clinicians should obtain a thorough history, including a family history of genetic diseases predisposing to intracranial vascular malformations. Moreover, they should also evaluate the temporal pattern of headaches, inquire about the associated symptoms, investigate vital signs, examine the patient for systemic or neurological signs, and perform a fundus examination to assess for abnormalities [10]. However, distinguishing between primary and secondary headaches is difficult, particularly in an ED setting [2]. Symptoms alone are inadequate criteria for differentiating between primary and secondary headaches because patients can experience a secondary headache with the same symptoms as any primary headache [11–13]. The diagnosis of secondary headaches can be suggested by the presence of red flags [14], which are clinical findings that point to a possible and serious cause of headaches. However, the presence of red flags does not always indicate underlying causes that require immediate treatment, potentially misleading clinicians to waste time and resources [15]. Therefore, many children with headaches undergo neuroimaging studies such as CT and MRI [16]. Brain MRI provides better visualization and essential information but is more expensive and may require sedation, especially in children under the age of six [17]. On the other hand, CT scans expose paediatric patients to radiation, increasing the risk of malignancy later in life [18,19]. Because of cranial bone marrow production, age-dependent risk is especially high in younger children [19,20].

When deciding whether to perform an imaging study in children with headaches, risk stratification based on clinical history and physical examination should be considered to ensure that the benefits of neuroimaging exceed the risks of radiation exposure from CT scans or sedation for MRI [21]. However, defining reliable red flags for the prediction of severe disorders and, consequently, validating criteria for the appropriate use of neuroimaging during diagnostic workup are challenging [22]. Many factors, such as teaching status, ownership, metropolitan area, insurance status, and ethnicity of patients, affect how frequently CT is used in various studies [23]. Among the studies reporting specialist consultations in patients with headaches admitted to the ED [24,25], only a few authors have considered the role of different specialists in ordering neuroimaging investigations in children with headaches [26].

The aim of our paper was to evaluate how specialist advice can influence the choice of neuroimaging studies in the paediatric ED.

2. Materials and Methods

This retrospective study included children with headaches admitted to the paediatric ED of Ospedale Maggiore Policlinico of Milano between January 2017 and January 2022. The same population was the subject of a recently published study approved by the ethics committee of our hospital [27]. The Inclusion criteria were age < 18 years, admission to the paediatric ED for headaches, and a lack of verbal or developmental delays. Patients who were unable to provide details about their headaches, such as the location or sudden onset, were excluded from this study. Very young children were also excluded unless their parents could provide such information. For patients who had more than one access to the ED due to headaches during the study period, only the most recent admission was considered.

The following data were evaluated for each patient: demographic characteristics, personal history of headache, clinical characteristics, underlying disorders, and the results of diagnostic procedures, including neuroimaging and laboratory testing. Headaches were classified into three categories: primary headaches (headaches without underlying medical conditions), secondary headaches (headaches associated with underlying medical conditions), and headaches of unknown aetiology. Secondary headaches were further grouped into intracranial (meningoencephalitis, cerebrovascular disorders, and structural abnormalities) and non-intracranial disorders (systemic infections, toxic-metabolic disorders, ocular diseases, otorhinolaryngological diseases, and functional disorders).

Medical consultations included visits to paediatricians, neurologists, and other specialists, such as otolaryngologists and ophthalmologists. The total number of consultations was recorded, as well as the various specialists involved. Furthermore, the number of neuroimaging investigations required by different specialists was assessed.

Excel was used for data collection, and statistical analysis was performed with R 4.3.0 (R Core Team Software, Vienna, Austria). Continuous variables were reported as mean and range values, while categorical variables were presented as frequencies and percentages. The Chi-square test or Fisher's exact test for small counts was used to compare the medical consulting and neuroimaging findings. Statistical significance was set at 5%.

3. Results

During the 5 years period of the study, 890 children with headaches were evaluated in our paediatric ED (mean age: 10.0 years; range: 1 to 17 years). The demographic data of the study population are summarized in Table 1. Most patients were discharged (90.8%, 808 patients), whereas the remaining patients were hospitalized (9.2%, 82 patients).

Table 1. Demographic data of 890 patients with headaches admitted to the ED.

Demographic Data		
Age (years)—mean (range)		10 (1–17)
Sex—N (%)	Male	430 (48.3)
	Female	460 (51.7)
Pre-existing headache—N (%) (881/890, 99.0%)	Yes	316 (35.9)
	Primary headache	224 (70.9)
	Secondary headache	44 (13.9)
	Unknown headache	48 (15.2)
	No	565 (64.1)
Underlying conditions—N (%)	No	795 (89.3)
	Systemic diseases	50 (5.6)
	Genetic neurological diseases	17 (1.9)
	Acquired neurological diseases	28 (3.1)

All patients underwent paediatric visits by the ED paediatricians. Overall, 261 specialist consultations were requested in the ED, including 240 neurological (92.0%),

46 ophthalmological (18.0%), and 20 otorhinolaryngologists (7.7%) consultations. Two specialist consultations were requested for 46 patients (17.6%), whereas only 1 patient (0.4%) received all three consultations (Table 2).

Table 2. Number of medical consultations.

Medical Consultations	Total Number (%)
Paediatrician	890 (100.0)
Paediatrician only	629 (70.7)
Specialist	261 (29.3)
Neurological	240 (92.0)
Otorhinolaryngological	20 (7.7)
Ophthalmological	46 (17.6)

Headaches were located frontotemporally in 611 patients (68.7%), occipital in 52 (5.8%), diffuse in 107 (12.0%), and unspecified in 120 (13.5%).

Primary headaches occurred in 337 (37.9%) patients, secondary headaches in 353 (39.7%) patients, and headaches of unknown aetiology in 200 (22.5%). Primary headache was diagnosed by paediatricians and neurologists in 43.5% and 56.5% of the patients, respectively. Paediatricians diagnosed secondary headaches in 65.6% of cases (intracranial diseases in 16 patients and non-intracranial disorders in 26 patients), whereas neurologists diagnosed secondary headaches in 34.4% of cases (intracranial diseases in 9 patients and non-intracranial disorders in 13 patients). All patients with headaches of unknown aetiology were visited by paediatricians and neurologists.

Overall, 173 neuroimaging examinations were performed, with 89 scans ordered by a paediatrician (51.4%) and 84 by a neurologist (48.6%). In particular, paediatricians required 81 out of 132 brain CT scans (61.4%), while neurologists ordered 23 out of 25 brain MRIs (92.0%). Both CT and MRI were performed in 16 patients, and most scans (62.5%) were ordered by neurologists (Table 3). Abnormalities were found in 27 of the 173 neuroimaging examinations performed (15.6%).

Table 3. Number of neuroimaging investigations according to medical consultations.

	Patients with Imaging N (%) (n = 173)	Brain CT N (%) (n = 132)	Brain MRI N (%) (n = 25)	Brain CT + MRI N (%) (n = 16)	p
Paediatrician	89 (51.4)	81 (61.4)	2 (8.0)	6 (37.5)	<0.001
Neurologist	84 (48.6)	51 (38.6)	23 (92.0)	10 (62.5)	

Legend. The p-value refers to the result of the Fisher exact test applied to the 2×3 contingency table obtained by comparing the variables "medical consultations" (paediatrician, neurologist) and "neuroimaging" (brain CT, brain MRI, brain CT + MRI).

4. Discussion

Neurological disorders represent a relevant component of paediatric emergencies, involving up to 20 to 40% of children with the highest severity codes at triage evaluation in the paediatric ED [28]. Epileptic and non–epileptic events and headaches account for over two–thirds of the cases [22]. In certain centers, over the last decade, the rate of paediatric ED visits for non–traumatic headaches has increased from 63.6 to 166% [29,30]. The high frequency of emergency clinical presentations is associated with an increasing need for specialized neuropaediatric consultants [22]. Consultations with specialists in ED are required for safe and effective patient care [31]. This process should result in a variety of outcomes, including the completion of procedures or investigations, as well as hospitalization or discharge [32–35]. Some studies have reported specialist consultations in patients with headaches admitted to the ED [24,25]. Still, only a few authors have investigated the role of different specialists in ordering neuroimaging investigations for children with headaches [26].

Our study showed that emergency paediatricians were the sole clinicians in charge of most children with headaches admitted to the ED, with specialist consultations required in only approximately one–third of the cases. This finding is consistent with those reported in other Italian studies, in which the rate of specialist visits ranged from 28.2% to 49.7% [24,25]. Therefore, we cannot exclude the possibility that the hospital's organization, patient triage method, and intra–hospital protocols used in our country played a role in explaining these results. According to the literature, most secondary headaches in our patients were benign and self-limiting [2,3,24,26,36–38], and they were usually managed by ED paediatricians. Nonetheless, paediatricians were also frequently involved in the diagnosis of headaches associated with intracranial disorders, whereas neurologists were most often responsible for the diagnosis of primary headaches. This finding could be partially explained by the difficulty of establishing a definitive diagnosis in children during their first visit because the diagnosis of primary headache is easily made when certain International Headache Society (IHS) criteria are fulfilled [39].

The first step in the evaluation of a child or adolescent with a headache is to distinguish between primary and secondary headaches [21]. Although most childhood headaches are benign, parents are frequently concerned about the possibility of a brain tumour or vascular malformation, especially if there is a family history of congenital aneurysms [17]. Clinicians should obtain detailed clinical history and perform comprehensive clinical examinations. The presence of provoking factors associated with migraine or tension-type headache, such as stress or sleep deprivation, as well as recent head trauma, fever, or features associated with systemic disease, suggesting secondary headaches, should be considered in the clinical history [5]. It is essential to evaluate the temporal pattern of headaches because acute or chronic progressive headaches are usually associated with secondary disorders. In contrast, episodic or chronic nonprogressive headaches may suggest a primary headache [40].

Family history should be investigated for the presence of primary or secondary headaches in other family members, including brain tumours, vascular disorders, and autoimmune diseases [5]. In all patients with headaches, detailed general and neurological examinations should be performed, including a search for meningismus, assessment of the cranial nerves, and examination of the optic discs [5,41,42]. Symptoms alone cannot distinguish between primary and secondary headaches since patients with secondary headaches may experience the same symptoms as those with primary headaches [11–13]. Nonetheless, the main goal of the clinical history and examination is to look for "red flags" [21], which are clinical findings that point to a possible and serious cause of headaches, compelling physicians to perform advanced investigations [15]. Certain red flags are more common in patients with secondary headaches [43], and patients with one or more red flags are at a higher risk of underlying intracranial diseases [39]. The main red flags included the following findings: (1) abnormal neurologic examination; (2) associated symptoms such as vertigo, intractable vomiting, mental status changes, focal neurologic signs, or systemic symptoms; (3) headache waking the child from sleep; (4) occipital headache; (5) first or worst headache; (6) recent headache of less than 6 months duration; (7) change in type of headache; (8) subacute onset and progressive headache; (9) new-onset headache in a child with immunosuppression; and (10) no family history of migraine or primary headaches. Although red flags act as screening tools that help physicians identify those patients with headaches who would benefit from immediate neuroimaging [44], they do not always indicate that the underlying cause requires emergency treatment [15]. Among the cases requiring specialist consultation, we found that neurologists were involved in over 90% of the cases, which is consistent with the results of other studies on headaches, in which the neurologist was the most frequently consulted specialist [25,26]. In a study of adults admitted to the ED for headaches by Relja et al., neurological visits accounted for 81.2% of specialist consultations and 12.7% of all neurological consultation visits to the ED during the same period [25]. In a study of 1833 patients admitted to the paediatric ED with headache, Rossi et al. requested 390 specialist consultation visits, including 187 neurological, 156 ophthalmological, 19 neurosurgical, and 28 otorhinolaryngologic consultations [26]. Headache is one of the main reasons for requiring an urgent neurological visit to the paediatric ED [25], and patients admitted to the ED for headaches have a high chance of being diagnosed with a secondary disorder [26]. The rarity of ophthalmologic and otorhinolaryngological consultations in our ED seems to be consistent with those of other studies [24,26]. Since headaches caused by ophthalmological problems are more frequently chronic, they are less common in emergency settings [24]. Although otorhinolaryngological consultation may be necessary if recurrent and chronic sinusitis is suspected [44], a diagnosis of acute uncomplicated sinusitis should be based solely on the clinical history and physical examination without the need for imaging [21].

Previous studies have reported that 6.3% to 44% of children admitted to the ED with headaches undergo neuroimaging studies [3,24,45–49]. The wide range of imaging rates reflects a lack of agreement or formal recommendations on the management of children and adolescents with headaches in the ED [26]. The decision to order imaging studies for children with headaches should involve risk stratification based on clinical history and physical examination to assess the benefits and risks of neuroimaging [21].

Brain CT is highly sensitive for detecting intracranial hemorrhage but less sensitive for evaluating intracranial masses and infections. Therefore, CT is appropriate for sudden severe headaches because their aetiology might be related to a ruptured aneurysm or arteriovenous malformation [50–52]. However, because brain CT exposes paediatric patients to radiation, increasing the risk of malignancy later in life [18,19], its use is restricted to specific cases [21]. Although brain MRI is the preferred neuroimaging technique for children and adolescents due to the lack of radiation exposure, it is not without risks, such as sedation or general anaesthesia [21]. Since headache is the only symptom of 1% of paediatric brain abnormalities [53–56], neuroimaging is considered unnecessary in patients with headaches who have no other neurologic symptoms, suggesting a serious intracranial disorder [54,57]. Nonetheless, overuse of CT [58] and MRI in paediatric ED has been reported, and there is a need for current studies covering paediatric imaging overuse trends, usage variability, and adherence to clinical protocols [59]. Although the American Academy of Neurology (AAN) Practice Guidelines recommended a diagnostic approach for children and adolescents with recurrent headaches, they made no specific statement about patients admitted to the ED for headaches [50].

Our study showed no significant difference in the number of neuroimaging studies required by paediatricians and neurologists. In contrast, Rossi et al. reported that emergency paediatricians ordered 63.5% of the neuroimaging investigations required for headaches in paediatrics, a neurologist ordered 30.4%, and another consultant ordered 4.8% [26]. However, we found that brain CT was most often ordered by the paediatricians and MRI by the neurologists. The outcomes observed in our study can be explained by several factors. First, in an emergency situation, paediatrician must quickly rule out life-threatening conditions that are frequently detected on brain CT scans. CT can be useful in this setting because it does not require sedation and is faster for acquiring brain images, although radiation exposure from CT scans in childhood has been linked to an increased risk of leukemia and brain tumors [19].

Second, even though brain MRI use in the emergency setting has recently increased due to the desire to provide radiation-free imaging, performing an MRI in the paediatric ED is still uncommon due to the need for sedation in very young children [60]. It is interesting to note that in paediatric patients with recurrent headache, provider specialty was associated with the likelihood of receiving a CT scan, with a neurologist being associated with a lower likelihood of a child undergoing a CT scan than a family physician [60].

Despite the fact that many patients have been seen by a paediatric neurologist, the frequency of headaches of unknown origin is high in our study. Indeed, we defined our cohort based on the primary discharge diagnosis without a specific follow-up program for these patients, which could have been useful for reclassifying headaches of unknown aetiology.

5. Conclusions

The diagnostic dilemma in evaluating children and adolescents with headaches is that most do not have intracranial disorders. Still, a small percentage of serious disease disorders may manifest clinically as isolated headaches. Therefore, many paediatric patients undergo brain CT and MRI scans [16]. Since CT uses ionizing radiation at doses that predispose patients, especially children, to malignancies [19], clinicians should weigh the risk of causing harm against the possibility of missing a serious disorder [61]. Reducing radiation exposure during the treatment of common diseases is a priority in the ED [62,63]. There are ongoing efforts to reduce radiation exposure through age and weight adjustments, as well as novel CT technologies [64].

Nonetheless, ED clinicians should use patient history or physical examination findings to establish the risk of an emergent intracranial abnormality in a child with a headache and to decide whether to order emergent brain imaging [50,51,65–69]. Several clinical evidence-based guidelines for children with headaches can help identify the patients who are more likely to have serious underlying causes for their headaches [16]. Although practice guidelines can be effective, they are not universally adopted, and the risk of missing an intracranial lesion persists even when followed [61]. Brain MRI use and availability in the ED have increased in recent years due to the desire to use radiation-free imaging [70] and reduce the length of stay in the ED until MRI imaging becomes available [60]. MRI techniques are evolving to detect intracranial disorders in children without exposing them to radiation risks, and rapid-sequence brain MRI protocols have been developed for paediatric patients [62,71].

The novelty of our study lies in defining the role of specialist consultations in the management of childhood headaches in the ED. Children with headaches admitted to the ED are first examined by a paediatrician, who is ultimately responsible for deciding whether to perform neuroimaging studies. The emergency paediatrician prefers brain CT to rule out life-threatening intracranial disorders in emergency settings. Neurologic consultation may be more useful in the diagnosis of primary or secondary headaches associated with a normal CT scan. In recent years, there has been a trend toward more conservative use of CT imaging in an attempt to limit paediatric patients' exposure to ionizing radiation [63]. A closer collaboration between emergency paediatricians and other ED specialists could improve this outcome.

Author Contributions: Conceptualization, A.M.C.; methodology, A.M.C.; formal analysis, M.T.M.; investigation, A.M.C., and G.B. (Gaia Bruschi), G.B.B. and G.B. (Giuseppe Bertolozzi); data curation, M.T.M.; writing—original draft preparation, A.M.C., and G.B. (Gaia Bruschi) and G.B.B.; writing—review, and editing, A.M.C. and G.B. (Giuseppe Bertolozzi). All authors have read and agreed to the published version of the manuscript.

Funding: This study was supported by the Ricerca Corrente grant (IRCCS RC-2023 Grant No. 01) from the Italian Ministry of Health.

Institutional Review Board Statement: The population reported in this study was recently published in a study approved by the Ethics Committee of Fondazione IRCCS Cà Granda Ospedale Maggiore Policlinico, 17 September 2022. This was the second analysis of the data from patients included in the Institutional Review Board Statement obtained from a previously published study.

Informed Consent Statement: The patients' written consent forms were not required owing to the retrospective nature of the study.

Data Availability Statement: The data presented in this study are available upon request from the corresponding author.

Acknowledgments: We thank A. Salici and A. Tirozzi for their contributions to data collection.

Conflicts of Interest: The authors declare no conflict of interest.

References

1. Sillanpaa, M.; Abu-Arafeh, I. Epidemiology of recurrent headache in children. In *Childhood Headache*; MacKeith Press: London, UK, 2002; pp. 19–34.
2. Conicella, E.; Raucci, U.; Vanacore, N.; Vigevano, F.; Reale, A.; Pirozzi, N.; Valeriani, M. The child with headache in a pediatric emergency department. *Headache* **2008**, *48*, 1005–1011. [CrossRef] [PubMed]
3. Kan, L.; Nagelberg, J.; Maytal, J. Headaches in a pediatric emergency department: Etiology, imaging, and treatment. *Headache* **2000**, *40*, 25–29. [CrossRef] [PubMed]
4. May, A. Hints on Diagnosing and Treating Headache. *Dtsch. Arztebl. Int.* **2018**, *115*, 299–308. [CrossRef] [PubMed]
5. Kelly, M.; Strelzik, J.; Langdon, R.; DiSabella, M. Pediatric headache: Overview. *Curr. Opin. Pediatr.* **2018**, *30*, 748–754. [CrossRef] [PubMed]
6. Özge, A.; Abu-Arafeh, I.; Gelfand, A.A.; Goadsby, P.J.; Cuvellier, J.C.; Valeriani, M.; Sergeev, A.; Barlow, K.; Uludüz, D.; Yalın, O.Ö.; et al. Experts' opinion about the pediatric secondary headaches diagnostic criteria of the ICHD-3 beta. *J. Headache Pain* **2017**, *18*, 113. [CrossRef]
7. Torriero, R.; Capuano, A.; Mariani, R.; Frusciante, R.; Tarantino, S.; Papetti, L.; Vigevano, F.; Valeriani, M. Diagnosis of primary headache in children younger than 6 years: A clinical challenge. *Cephalalgia* **2017**, *37*, 947–954. [CrossRef] [PubMed]
8. Celle, M.E.; Carelli, V.; Fornarino, S. Secondary headache in children. *Neurol. Sci.* **2010**, *31*, S81–S82. [CrossRef]
9. Lewis, D.W.; Qureshi, F. Acute headache in children and adolescents presenting to the emergency department. *Headache* **2000**, *40*, 200–203. [CrossRef]
10. Yonker, M. Secondary Headaches in Children and Adolescents: What Not to Miss. *Curr. Neurol. Neurosci. Rep.* **2018**, *18*, 61. [CrossRef]
11. Cady, R.K. Red flags and comfort signs for ominous secondary headaches. *Otolaryngol. Clin. N. Am.* **2014**, *47*, 289–299. [CrossRef]
12. Schankin, C.J.; Straube, A. Secondary headaches: Secondary or still primary? *J. Headache Pain* **2012**, *13*, 263–270. [CrossRef] [PubMed]
13. Ravishankar, K. Optimising primary headache management. *J. Assoc. Physicians India* **2006**, *54*, 928–934. [PubMed]
14. García-Azorín, D.; Abelaira-Freire, J.; González-García, N.; Rodriguez-Adrada, E.; Schytz, H.W.; Barloese, M.; Guerrero, Á.L.; Porta-Etessam, J.; Martín-Sánchez, F.J. Sensitivity of the SNNOOP10 list in the high-risk secondary headache detection. *Cephalalgia* **2022**, *42*, 1521–1531. [CrossRef] [PubMed]
15. Yayıcı Köken, Ö.; Danış, A.; Yüksel, D.; Aksoy, A.; Öztoprak, Ü.; Aksoy, E. Pediatric headache: Are the red flags misleading or prognostic? *Brain Dev.* **2021**, *43*, 372–379. [CrossRef]
16. Trofimova, A.; Vey, B.L.; Mullins, M.E.; Wolf, D.S.; Kadom, N. Imaging of Children with Nontraumatic Headaches. *AJR Am. J. Roentgenol.* **2018**, *210*, 8–17. [CrossRef] [PubMed]
17. Alexiou, G.A.; Argyropoulou, M.I. Neuroimaging in childhood headache: A systematic review. *Pediatr. Radiol.* **2013**, *43*, 777–784. [CrossRef] [PubMed]
18. Trottier, E.D.; Bailey, B.; Lucas, N.; Lortie, A. Diagnosis of migraine in the pediatric emergency department. *Pediatr. Neurol.* **2013**, *49*, 40–45. [CrossRef]
19. Pearce, M.S.; Salotti, J.A.; Little, M.P.; McHugh, K.; Lee, C.; Kim, K.P.; Howe, N.L.; Ronckers, C.M.; Rajaraman, P.; Sir Craft, A.W.; et al. Radiation exposure from CT scans in childhood and subsequent risk of leukaemia and brain tumours: A retrospective cohort study. *Lancet* **2012**, *4*, 499–505. [CrossRef]
20. Alzen, G.; Benz-Bohm, G. Radiation protection in pediatric radiology. *Dtsch. Arztebl. Int.* **2011**, *108*, 407–414. [CrossRef]
21. Camargo, A.; Kanekar, S. Neuroimaging in Pediatric Headache. *Neurol. Clin.* **2022**, *40*, 679–698. [CrossRef]
22. Mastrangelo, M.; Baglioni, V. Management of Neurological Emergencies in Children: An Updated Overview. *Neuropediatrics* **2021**, *52*, 242–251. [CrossRef] [PubMed]
23. Hoshiko, S.; Smith, D.; Fan, C.; Jones, C.R.; McNeel, S.V.; Cohen, R.A. Trends in CT scan rates in children and pregnant women: Teaching, private, public and nonprofit facilities. *Pediatr. Radiol.* **2014**, *44*, 522–528. [CrossRef] [PubMed]
24. Scagni, P.; Pagliero, R. Headache in an Italian pediatric emergency department. *J. Headache Pain* **2008**, *9*, 83–87. [CrossRef] [PubMed]
25. Relja, G.; Granato, A.; Capozzoli, F.; Maggiore, C.; Catalan, M.; Pizzolato, G.; Zalukar, W.; Livia, V.; Gregorutti, S.; Zorzon, M. Nontraumatic headache in the Emergency Department: A survey in the province of Trieste. *J. Headache Pain* **2005**, *6*, 298–300. [CrossRef] [PubMed]
26. Rossi, R.; Versace, A.; Lauria, B.; Grasso, G.; Castagno, E.; Ricceri, F.; Pagliero, R.; Urbino, A.F. Headache in the pediatric emergency department: A 5-year retrospective study. *Cephalalgia* **2018**, *38*, 1765–1772. [CrossRef] [PubMed]
27. Cappellari, A.M.; Margiotta, S.; Bruschi, G.; Alicandro, G.; Castellazzi, M.L.; Rocchi, A.; Venturelli, E.; Bertolozzi, G. Impact of COVID-19 Pandemic on Headache Evaluations in the Pediatric Emergency Department. *Pediatr. Neurol.* **2022**, *137*, 49–53. [CrossRef]
28. Palmieri, A.; Dau, D.; Gallarotti, F.; Pavanello, M.; Di Pietro, P. Neurological disorders in a pediatric emergency room: Epidemiology and clinical aspects. *Minerva Pediatr.* **2006**, *58*, 289–297. (In Italian) [PubMed]
29. Vetri, L.; Messina, L.M.; Drago, F.; D'Aiuto, F.; Vanadia, F.; Brighina, F.; Raieli, V. Are paediatric headaches in the emergency department increasing? An Italian experience. *Funct. Neurol.* **2019**, *34*, 188–195.

30. Perry, M.C.; Yaeger, S.K.; Toto, R.L.; Suresh, S.; Hickey, R.W. A Modern Epidemic: Increasing Pediatric Emergency Department Visits and Admissions for Headache. *Pediatr. Neurol.* **2018**, *89*, 19–25. [CrossRef]
31. Voaklander, B.; Gaudet, L.A.; Kirkland, S.W.; Keto-Lambert, D.; Villa-Roel, C.; Rowe, B.H. Interventions to improve consultations in the emergency department: A systematic review. *Acad. Emerg. Med.* **2022**, *29*, 1475–1495. [CrossRef]
32. Brick, C.; Lowes, J.; Lovstrom, L.; Kokotilo, A.; Villa-Roel, C.; Lee, P.; Lang, E.; Rowe, B.H. The impact of consultation on length of stay in tertiary care emergency departments. *Emerg. Med. J.* **2014**, *31*, 134–138. [CrossRef]
33. Rosen, P. Emergency department disposition and knowledge of other specialties. *J. Emerg. Med.* **1986**, *4*, 325–326. [CrossRef] [PubMed]
34. Tintinalli, J.; McCall, K. Importance of emergency physicians as referral sources for academic medical centers. *Ann. Emerg. Med.* **1994**, *23*, 65–69. [CrossRef] [PubMed]
35. Lee, R.; Woods, R.; Bullard, M.; Holroyd, B.R.; Rowe, B.H. Consultations in emergency medicine: A systematic review of the literature. *Emerg. Med. J.* **2008**, *25*, 4–9. [CrossRef] [PubMed]
36. Lewis, D.W. Headache in the pediatric emergency department. *Semin. Pediatr. Neurol.* **2001**, *8*, 46–51. [CrossRef] [PubMed]
37. Hsiao, H.J.; Huang, J.L.; Hsia, S.H.; Lin, J.J.; Huang, I.A.; Wu, C.T. Headache in the pediatric emergency service: A medical center experience. *Pediatr. Neonatol.* **2014**, *55*, 208–212. [CrossRef]
38. Gupta, V.; Khandelwal, N.; Prabhakar, A.; Satish Kumar, A.; Ahuja, C.K.; Singh, P. Prevalence of normal head CT and positive CT findings in a large cohort of patients with chronic headaches. *Neuroradiol. J.* **2015**, *28*, 421–425. [CrossRef] [PubMed]
39. Roser, T.; Bonfert, M.; Ebinger, F.; Blankenburg, M.; Ertl-Wagner, B.; Heinen, F. Primary versus secondary headache in children: A frequent diagnostic challenge in clinical routine. *Neuropediatrics* **2013**, *44*, 34–39. [CrossRef]
40. Blume, H.K. Childhood headache: A brief review. *Pediatr. Ann.* **2017**, *46*, e155–e165. [CrossRef]
41. Headache Classification Committee of the International Headache Society (IHS). The International Classification of Headache Disorders. *Cephalalgia* **2018**, *38*, 1–211. [CrossRef]
42. Hershey, A.D. Pediatric headache. *Continuum* **2015**, *21*, 1132–1145. [CrossRef]
43. Park, E.G.; Yoo, I.H. The diagnostic values of red flags in pediatric patients with headache. *Brain Dev.* **2022**, *44*, 512–519. [CrossRef] [PubMed]
44. Sobri, M.; Lamont, A.C.; Alias, N.A.; Win, M.N. Red flags in patients presenting with headache: Clinical indications for neuroimaging. *Br. J. Radiol.* **2003**, *76*, 532–535. [CrossRef]
45. Cain, M.R.; Arkilo, D.; Linabery, A.M.; Kharbanda, A.B. Emergency Department Use of Neuroimaging in Children and Adolescents Presenting with Headache. *J. Pediatr.* **2018**, *201*, 196–201. [CrossRef] [PubMed]
46. Burton, L.J.; Quinn, B.; Pratt-Cheney, J.L.; Pourani, M. Headache etiology in a pediatric emergency department. *Pediatr. Emerg. Care* **1997**, *13*, 1–4. [CrossRef] [PubMed]
47. Eapen, A.; Sivaswamy, L.; Agarwal, R.; Thomas, R. Management of pediatric migraine in a tertiary care versus community based emergency department: An observational pilot study. *Pediatr. Neurol.* **2014**, *50*, 164–170. [CrossRef] [PubMed]
48. Lateef, T.M.; Grewal, M.; McClintock, W.; Chamberlain, J.; Kaulas, H.; Nelson, K.B. Headache in young children in the emergency department: Use of computed tomography. *Pediatrics* **2009**, *124*, e12–e17. [CrossRef]
49. Richer, L.; Graham, L.; Klassen, T.; Rowe, B. Emergency department management of acute migraine in children in Canada: A practice variation study. *Headache* **2007**, *47*, 703–710. [CrossRef]
50. Lewis, D.W.; Ashwal, S.; Dahl, G.; Dorbad, D.; Hirtz, D.; Prensky, A.; Jarjour, I.; Quality Standards Subcommittee of the American Academy of Neurology; Practice Committee of the Child Neurology Society. Practice parameter: Evaluation of children and adolescents with recurrent headaches. Report of the Quality Standards Subcommittee of the American Academy of Neurology and the Practice Committee of the Child Neurology Society. *Neurology* **2002**, *59*, 490–498. [CrossRef]
51. Hayes, L.L.; Palasis, S.; Bartel, T.B.; Booth, T.N.; Iyer, R.S.; Jones, J.Y.; Kadom, N.; Milla, S.S.; Myseros, J.S.; Pakalnis, A.; et al. ACR appropriateness criteria Headache–child. *J. Am. Coll. Radiol.* **2018**, *15*, S78–S90. [CrossRef]
52. Mortimer, A.M.; Bradley, M.D.; Stoodley, N.G.; Renowden, S.A. Thunderclap headache: Diagnostic considerations and neuroimaging features. *Clin. Radiol.* **2013**, *68*, e101–e113. [CrossRef] [PubMed]
53. Larson, D.B.; Johnson, L.W.; Schnell, B.M.; Goske, M.J.; Salisbury, S.R.; Forman, H.P. Rising use of CT in child visits to the emergency department in the United States, 1995–2008. *Radiology* **2011**, *259*, 793–801. [CrossRef] [PubMed]
54. Dooley, J.M. The evaluation and management of pediatric headaches. *Paediatr. Child Health* **2009**, *14*, 24–30. [CrossRef] [PubMed]
55. DeVries, A.; Young, P.C.; Wall, E.; Getchius, T.S.; Li, C.H.; Whitney, J.; Rosenberg, A. CT scan utilization patterns in pediatric patients with recurrent headache. *Pediatrics* **2013**, *132*, e1–e8. [CrossRef] [PubMed]
56. Ahmed, M.A.; Martinez, A.; Cahill, D.; Chong, K.; Whitehouse, W.P. When to image neurologically normal children with headaches: Development of a decision rule. *Acta Paediatr.* **2010**, *99*, 940–943. [CrossRef] [PubMed]
57. Raucci, U.; Della Vecchia, N.; Ossella, C.; Paolino, M.C.; Villa, M.P.; Reale, A.; Parisi, P. Management of Childhood Headache in the Emergency Department. Review of the Literature. *Front. Neurol.* **2019**, *23*, 886. [CrossRef] [PubMed]
58. Brenner, D.J.; Hall, E.J. Computed tomography—An increasing source of radiation exposure. *N. Engl. J. Med.* **2007**, *357*, 2277–2284. [CrossRef] [PubMed]
59. Ohana, O.; Soffer, S.; Zimlichman, E.; Klang, E. Overuse of CT and MRI in paediatric emergency departments. *Br. J. Radiol.* **2018**, *91*, 20170434. [CrossRef]

60. Scheinfeld, M.H.; Moon, J.Y.; Fagan, M.J.; Davoudzadeh, R.; Wang, D.; Taragin, B.H. MRI usage in a pediatric emergency department: An analysis of usage and usage trends over 5 years. *Pediatr. Radiol.* **2017**, *47*, 327–332. [CrossRef]
61. Wylie, M.C.; Merritt, C.; Clark, M.; Garro, A.C.; Rutman, M.S. Imaging of pediatric head injury in the emergency department. *Pediatr. Emerg. Care* **2014**, *30*, 680–685. [CrossRef]
62. Willis, C.E.; Slovis, T.L. The ALARA concept in pediatric CR and DR: Dose reduction in pediatric radiographic exams—A white paper conference executive summary. *Pediatr. Radiol.* **2004**, *34*, S162–S164. [CrossRef] [PubMed]
63. Frush, D.P.; Frush, K.S. The ALARA concept in pediatric imaging: Building bridges between radiology and emergency medicine: Consensus conference on imaging safety and quality for children in the emergency setting, Feb. 23–24, 2008, Orlando, FL—Executive Summary. *Pediatr. Radiol.* **2008**, *38*, S629–S632. [CrossRef] [PubMed]
64. Callahan, M.J. CT dose reduction in practice. *Pediatr. Radiol.* **2011**, *41*, 488–492. [CrossRef] [PubMed]
65. Lewis, D.W.; Koch, T. Headache evaluation in children and adolescents: When to worry? When to scan? *Pediatr. Ann.* **2010**, *39*, 399–406. [CrossRef] [PubMed]
66. Gofshteyn, J.S.; Stephenson, D.J. Diagnosis and Management of Childhood Headache. *Curr. Probl. Pediatr. Adolesc. Health Care* **2016**, *46*, 36–51. [CrossRef] [PubMed]
67. Tsze, D.S.; Ochs, J.B.; Gonzalez, A.E.; Dayan, P.S. Red flag findings in children with headaches: Prevalence and association with emergency department neuroimaging. *Cephalalgia* **2019**, *39*, 185–196. [CrossRef] [PubMed]
68. Kabbouche, M.A.; Cleves, C. Evaluation and management of children and adolescents presenting with an acute setting. *Semin. Pediatr. Neurol.* **2010**, *17*, 105–108. [CrossRef]
69. Detsky, M.E.; McDonald, D.R.; Baerlocher, M.O.; Tomlinson, G.A.; McCrory, D.C.; Booth, C.M. Does this patient with headache have a migraine or need neuroimaging? *JAMA* **2006**, *296*, 1274–1283. [CrossRef]
70. Goske, M.J.; Applegate, K.E.; Boylan, J.; Butler, P.F.; Callahan, M.J.; Coley, B.D.; Farley, S.; Frush, D.P.; Hernanz-Schulman, M.; Jaramillo, D.; et al. The image gently campaign: Working together to change practice. *AJR Am. J. Roentgenol.* **2008**, *190*, 273–274. [CrossRef]
71. Penzkofer, A.K.; Pfluger, T.; Pochmann, Y.; Meissner, O.; Leinsinger, G. MR imaging of the brain in pediatric patients: Diagnostic value of HASTE sequences. *AJR Am. J. Roentgenol.* **2002**, *179*, 509–514. [CrossRef]

children

MDPI

Communication

High CCL2 Levels Detected in CSF of Patients with Pediatric Pseudotumor Cerebri Syndrome

Jacob Genizi [1,2,*], Lotan Berger [1], Muhammad Mahajnah [2,3], Yulia Shlonsky [4], Orit Golan-Shany [4], Azriel Romem [1], Ayelet Halevy [5], Keren Nathan [1], Rajech Sharkia [6,7], Abdelnaser Zalan [7], Aharon Kessel [2,8] and Rony Cohen [5,9]

1 Pediatric Department, Bnai Zion Medical Center, Haifa 3104802, Israel; lotan269@gmail.com (L.B.); azrikel@gmail.com (A.R.); keren.nathan@b-zion.org.il (K.N.)
2 Bruce Rappaport Faulty of Medicine, Technion, Haifa 3109601, Israel; muhamadmah@hymc.gov.il (M.M.); aharon.kessel@b-zion.org.il (A.K.)
3 Pediatric Neurology Unit, Hillel Yaffe Medical Center, Hadera 3810000, Israel
4 Microbiology Lab, Bnai Zion Medical Center, Haifa 3104802, Israel; yulia.shlonsky@b-zion.org.il (Y.S.); orit.golan-shany@b-zion.org.il (O.G.-S.)
5 Department of Pediatric Neurology, Schneider Children's Medical Center of Israel, Petah Tikva 4920235, Israel; drayelethalevy@gmail.com (A.H.); drcohenrony@gmail.com (R.C.)
6 Beit-Berl Academic College, Beit-Berl 4490500, Israel; rajachsharkia@hotmail.com
7 Unit of Human Biology and Genetics, Triangle Regional Research and Development Center, Kfar Qari' 3007500, Israel; dr.zalan@hotmail.com
8 Division of Allergy and Clinical Immunology, Bnai Zion Medical Center, Haifa 3104802, Israel
9 Faculty of Medicine, Tel Aviv University, Tel Aviv 6997801, Israel
* Correspondence: genizij@gmail.com; Tel.: +972-4-8359662; Fax: +972-4-8359675

Abstract: Pseudotumor cerebri (PTC) is a disorder characterized by increased intracranial pressure in the absence of a structural lesion or other identifiable cause. Cytokines, which are involved in the regulation of immune responses and inflammation, have been implicated in the pathogenesis of PTC. In a prospective, cross-sectional study at three centers in Israel, we analyzed cerebrospinal fluid (CSF) samples from 60 children aged 0.5–18 years, including 43 children with a definitive diagnosis of PTC and a control group of 17 children. Levels of IL-4, IL-10, IL-17, CCL2, CCL7, CCL8, CCL13, BDNF, and IFN-γ were measured using ELISA kits. Levels of CCL2 were significantly higher in the PTC group compared to the control group ($p < 0.05$), with no other significant differences in the measured cytokines between the two groups. The groups did not differ significantly in clinical presentation, imaging, treatment, or ophthalmic findings. Our findings provide preliminary evidence that CCL2 may be involved in the pathogenesis of PTC and may serve a potential target for therapy in PTC.

Keywords: pseudotumor cerebri; cytokines; chemokines; etiology; pediatrics

1. Introduction

Pseudotumor cerebri (PTC) is a syndrome consisting of elevated intracranial pressure (250 mm water in adults and 280 mm water in sedated children), a chemically and hematologically normal cerebrospinal fluid (CSF) composition, and papilledema with occasional abducens nerve paresis [1]. PTC is diagnosed following the exclusion of secondary causes of elevated intracranial pressure, such as space-occupying lesions or venous sinus thrombosis, based on appropriate investigations, including brain imaging. The pathogenesis of the raised CSF pressure is still not clear. Some have proposed an increase in CSF production, impairment in CSF absorption, or cerebral edema [2–4]. Several studies have proposed that an inflammatory process is implicated in the pathogenesis of PTC [5–8]. Cytokines are glycoproteins that control inflammation. Elevated levels of inflammatory cytokines, including IL-6, IL-17, IL-1a, and CCL2, were found in a small group of PTC patients [5]. However, those results were inconclusive, requiring further work with a larger patient cohort. Accordingly, our study examined CSF levels of cytokines and chemokines in a larger group of pediatric patients with PTC matched to a control group.

2. Materials and Methods

2.1. Study Population and Procedure

A prospective, cross-sectional study was conducted in the pediatric departments of three medical centers in Israel: Bnei Zion, Schneider Children's, and Hillel Yaffe medical centers. Participants were children examined at the centers from 1 January 2020 to 30 December 2022. Children with pseudotumor cerebri, aged 0.5–18 years, were assigned to the study group (CSF was collected before treatment). Children whose clinical symptoms were consistent with increased intracranial pressure and who underwent lumbar puncture (LP), but where PTC was ruled out, served as a control group. An ophthalmologist and a pediatric neurologist conducted a thorough evaluation of all the children. The collected data included a wide range of information, such as clinical symptoms, imaging outcomes, treatment details, ophthalmic examination, and an analysis of the cerebrospinal fluid (CSF). Each hospital obtained its own ethical approval, and the caregivers of all participants provided written informed consent. The local Helsinki committee approved the study.

The CSF was investigated for the following cytokines: IL-4, IL-10, IL-17, CCL2, CCL7, CCL8, CCL13, BDNF, and IFN-γ. The samples were stored at a temperature of -80 degrees Celsius and analyzed at the end of the study. Samples were analyzed using the Luminex xMAP multiplex cytokine assay testing kit—a sandwich enzyme-linked immunosorbent assay (ELISA) kit.

2.2. Statistical Analyses

Patients with and without PTC were compared via the chi-square test or Fisher's exact test, where appropriate, for the categorical data and via independent t-tests for the continuous variables. Odds ratios and their 95% confidence intervals were computed. Significance was considered to be $p < 0.05$. Statistical analyses were performed using SPSS software version 21 (SPSS, Chicago, IL, USA).

3. Results

CSF samples from 60 children were collected. Forty three were diagnosed with pseudotumor cerebri, and the other seventeen children in the control group. The distinctive features of the two groups are outlined in Table 1. As noted above, patients in the control group had clinical symptoms consistent with increased intracranial pressure, but their LP opening pressure was normal. The patients in the control group had nonspecific headaches without a chronic headache syndrome or other chronic disease. The patient mean age was 11.8 in the study group and 11.4 in the control group, without statistical differences between them. Patients were more likely to be female, with a male/female ratios of 20/23 and 7/10 for the study group and control group, respectively, again, with no significant differences between them. Clinical symptoms also did not differ significantly between the groups. The opening pressure, as expected, was higher in the study group; please see Table 1.

Table 1. Characteristics of the study and control groups.

Characteristic	PTC Group (n = 43)	Control Group (n = 17)	p
Mean age	11.8 years	11.4 years	$p = 0.34$
Sex (male/female)	20/23	7/10	$p = 0.45$
Opening pressure (cm H_2O)	40	24	$p < 0.001$

The Luminex xMAP panel was run for IL-4, IL-10, IL-17, CCL2, CCL7, CCL8, CCL13, BDNF, and IFN-γ. Only CCL2 was detected in the CSF at significant levels, (Figure A1) and it was significantly higher (<0.03) in the PTC group compared to the control group (Table 2).

Table 2. Cytokine levels in CSF of PTC and control groups.

Cytokine	PTC Group (pg/mL)	Control Group (pg/mL)	p-Value
IL-10	<42.95	<42.95	0.62
IL-4	<21.59	<21.59	0.53
IL-17	<13.15	<13.15	0.58
CCL2	222	165.2	<0.03
CCL7	<33.85	<33.85	0.72
CCL8	<13.47	<13.47	0.55
CCL13	<5.51	<5.51	0.46
BDNF	<17.93	<17.93	0.48
IFN-γ	<9.78	<9.78	0.6

4. Discussion

We found significantly higher CCL2 levels in the CSF of the pediatric PTC group compared to the control group. This finding was consistent with Dhungana et al.'s [5] finding of increased CCL2 levels in the CSF of adult patients with PTC, based on a small study (eight PTC patients) and using a cytokine antibody array kit. However, they also reported elevated levels of CCL7 and CCL8. In our study, based on 47 pediatric patients with PTC and using a quantitative assay with ELISA, levels of CCL7 and CCL8 were not measurable. On the other hand, Ball et al. [9] found no differences in levels of either CCL2 or other cytokines (IL-1beta, IL-6, IL-8, TNF alpha, hepatocyte growth factor, nerve growth factor, and PAI-1) in patients with idiopathic intracranial hypertension compared to controls.

CCL2 is a chemokine that is involved in the recruitment of monocytes to sites of inflammation. CCL2 activates β1 integrins and regulates the adhesion and chemotaxis of macrophages [10]. Fibroblasts and epithelial cells have the capability to generate CCL2 as well. CCL2 plays a significant role in facilitating the infiltration of monocytes into tissues during inflammatory events. Its expression is induced in response to inflammatory triggers such as infection and tissue injury. The production of CCL2 has been observed in various TH1/M1 inflammatory disorders, including inflammatory diseases. Additionally, CCL2 production is recognized as a characteristic feature of TH2/M2 responses, and it enhances the production of TH2-type cytokines, particularly IL-4, through activated T cells [10]. In the context of PTC, it is thought to play a role in the recruitment of macrophages to the subarachnoid space, leading to inflammation and increased intracranial pressure. It has been suggested that CCL2 may be involved in the regulation of the blood–brain barrier and the production of CSF [11].

Edwards et al. [7], in a small (11 patients) study on adults with PTC, compared levels of IL-17, IL-10, IL-4, and IFN-γ among PTC patients and a control group of patients with other inflammatory diseases (chronic inflammatory demyelinating peripheral neuropathy (CIDP) and multiple sclerosis (MS)). IL-17 was detected among both some PTC patients and patients with MS, but levels of IL-10 were higher among MS patients compared to CIDP and PTC patients. IL-17 is a cytokine produced by T-helper 17 (Th17) cells. T-helper 17 cells play a crucial role in many inflammatory diseases and are involved in recruiting inflammatory cells to the CNS [12]. As such, they may be implicated in the development of PTC as well. IL-10 acts to limit CNS inflammation by modulating the sensitivity of resident glia and infiltrating leukocytes towards activating stimuli, as well as diminishing the production of inflammatory mediators [13]. However, in our study, we found no significant differences in levels of either IL-10 or IL-17 between the PTC and control groups.

We also found no differences in levels of brain-derived neurotrophic factor (BDNF) and IFN-γ between pediatric patients with PTC and the control group. BDNF plays a crucial role in the regulation of neuronal survival, structure, and function, particularly in brain regions responsible for intricate cognitive processes. Studies indicate that disruptions in the signaling pathway of BDNF may contribute to the cognitive deterioration seen in specific neuropsychiatric and inflammatory conditions [14]. Interferon-γ (IFN-γ) is a cytokine produced by T-helper 1 (Th1) cells [15]. Altıokka-Uzun et al. [16], studying adults with idiopathic intracranial hypertension, found elevated levels of TNF-α, IFN-γ, IL-4, IL-10, IL-12, and IL-17 in the CSF of study patients compared to controls. In our study, IL-4, IL-10, IL-17, BDNF, and IFN-γ were all undetected in the CSF of pediatric patients with PTC.

The differences between our findings and those of previous studies may be due to differences in patient populations—specifically, the fact that we looked at pediatric patients with PTC, while all other studies examined adults. There are some known differences between adult and pediatric PTC patients, mainly in the greater prevalence of the male sex and not being obese in young children [17].

The underlying causes of PTC remain undisclosed [18]. While transverse or sigmoid sinus stenosis or atrophy is commonly observed in PTC [1], it is likely a secondary effect rather than the primary cause, resulting from the increased pressure [19]. Nonetheless, stenosis can exacerbate intracranial pressure by impeding the proper removal of cerebrospinal fluid (CSF). The increased prevalence of obesity among PTC patients and the incidence of PTC after specific medicines [1] could potentially be attributed to the impact of estrogen or retinoic acid on epithelial cells, resulting in a reduced CSF outflow. Genetic investigations involving AQP4, which facilitates the movement of water in and out of the brain, have not found any relationship with PTC [20]. Other potential factors to consider include mild inflammation and dysfunction within the glymphatic pathway [21]. In a recent study [18], we explored the role of viruses in the pathogenesis of PTC, but found no supporting evidence. In the present study, we found evidence for a potential role of inflammation (CCL2) in the pathogenesis of PTC. This may support the use of anti-inflammatory therapies, including cytokine-targeted therapies, in the treatment of PTC.

4.1. Limitations

Our study, while larger than previous studies (e.g., [5]), was still relatively small, with a small control group; we also did not measure serum levels. We used ELISA, but CCL2 should be confirmed using other methods. Larger studies and ones measuring serum levels are warranted.

4.2. Conclusions

Our study provides preliminary evidence that CCL2 may be involved in the pathogenesis of PTC. Additional research is required to validate these findings and explore the therapeutic potential of cytokines as targets for PTC treatment.

Author Contributions: Conceptualization, J.G., M.M., A.H., K.N., A.K. and R.C.; Methodology, J.G., L.B., M.M., A.R., A.H., K.N., A.K. and R.C.; Validation, L.B., O.G.-S., A.R. and R.S.; Formal analysis, L.B., Y.S., O.G.-S. and A.Z.; Investigation, J.G., L.B., M.M., Y.S. and O.G.-S.; Resources, R.S. and A.Z.; Writing—original draft, J.G. and M.M.; Writing—review & editing, R.C.; Project administration, J.G. All authors have read and agreed to the published version of the manuscript.

Funding: This research was funded by the Israeli Pediatric Association and by limited internal resources from the Triangle Research and Development Center (TRDC).

Institutional Review Board Statement: Bnai Zion IRB # 0041-18 BNZ.

Informed Consent Statement: Informed consent was obtained from all subjects involved in the study.

Data Availability Statement: Data is unavailable due to privacy restrictions.

Conflicts of Interest: The authors declare no conflict of interest.

Appendix A

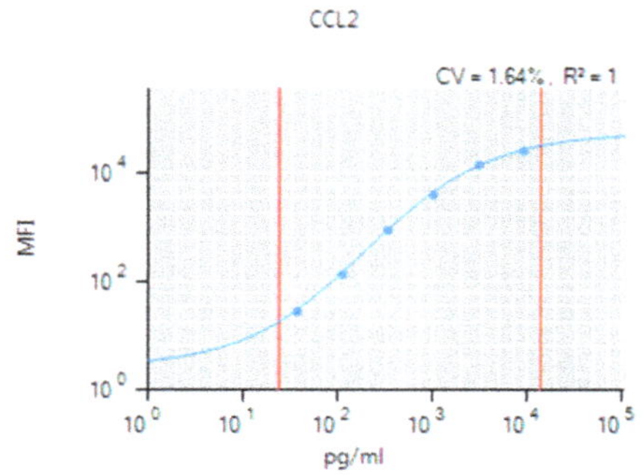

5-P.log(1.00, 10.84, 0.68, 5.26, 0.66)
DC = (23.52, 13,654) Chi = 0.048%

Figure A1. CCL2 Levels among PTC research group.

References

1. Friedman, D.I.; Jacobson, D.M. Diagnostic criteria for idiopathic intracranial hypertension. *Neurology* **2002**, *59*, 1492–1495. [CrossRef] [PubMed]
2. Sahs, A.L.; Joynt, R.J. Brain swelling of unknown cause. *Neurology* **1954**, *6*, 791–803. [CrossRef]
3. Johnston, I. Reduced CSF absorption syndrome. Reappraisal of benign intracranial hypertension and related conditions. *Lancet* **1973**, *2*, 418–421. [CrossRef] [PubMed]
4. King, J.O.; Mitchell, P.J.; Thompson, K.R.; Tress, B.M. Cerebral venography and manometry in idiopathic intracranial hypertension. *Neurology* **1995**, *45*, 2224–2228. [CrossRef]
5. Dhungana, S.; Sharrack, B.; Woodroofe, N. Cytokines and chemokines in idiopathic intracranial hypertension. *Headache* **2009**, *49*, 282–285. [CrossRef]
6. Dhungana, S.; Sharrack, B.; Woodroofe, N. IL-1β, TNF and IP-10 in the cerebrospinal fluid and serum are not altered in patients with idiopathic intracranial hypertension compared to controls. *Clin. Endocrinol.* **2009**, *71*, 896–897. [CrossRef]
7. Edwards, L.; Constantinescu, C. Cytokines in idiopathic intracranial hypertension CSF. *Headache* **2010**, *50*, 323–325.
8. Subramanian, P.; Goldenberg-Cohen, N.; Shukla, S.; Cheskin, L.; Miller, N. Plasma ghrelin levels are normal in obese patients with idiopathic intracranial hypertension (pseudotumor cerebri). *Am. J. Ophthalmol.* **2004**, *138*, 109–113. [CrossRef]
9. Ball, A.K.; Sinclair, A.J.; Curnow, S.J.; Tomlinson, J.W.; Burdon, M.A.; Walker, E.A.; Stewart, P.M.; Nightingale, P.G.; Clarke, C.E.; Rauz, S. Elevated cerebrospinal fluid (CSF) leptin in idiopathic intracranial hypertension (IIH): Evidence for hypothalamic leptin resistance? *Clin. Endocrinol.* **2009**, *70*, 863–869. [CrossRef]
10. Ashida, N.; Arai, H.; Yamasaki, M.; Kita, T. Differential signaling for MCP-1-dependent integrin activation and chemotaxis. *Ann. N. Y. Acad. Sci.* **2001**, *947*, 387–389. [CrossRef]
11. Dimitrijevic, O.B.; Stamatovic, S.M.; Keep, R.F.; Andjelkovic, A.V. Effects of the chemokine CCL2 on blood-brain barrier permeability during ischemia-reperfusion injury. *J. Cereb. Blood Flow Metab.* **2006**, *26*, 797–810. [CrossRef]
12. Rostami, A.; Ciric, B. Role of Th17 cells in the pathogenesis of CNS inflammatory demyelination. *J. Neurol. Sci.* **2013**, *333*, 76–87. [CrossRef] [PubMed]
13. Burmeister, A.R.; Marriott, I. The interleukin-10 family of cytokines and their role in the CNS. *Front. Cell. Neurosci.* **2018**, *12*, 458. [CrossRef] [PubMed]
14. Kauer-Sant'Anna, M.; Kapczinski, F.; Andreazza, A.C.; Bond, D.J.; Lam, R.W.; Young, L.T.; Yatham, L.N. Brain-derived neurotrophic factor and inflammatory markers in patients with early- vs. late-stage bipolar disorder. *Int. J. Neuropsychopharmacol.* **2009**, *12*, 447–458. [CrossRef] [PubMed]
15. Jorgovanovic, D.; Song, M.; Wang, L.; Zhang, Y. Roles of IFN-γ in tumor progression and regression: A review. *Biomark. Res.* **2020**, *8*, 49. [CrossRef] [PubMed]
16. Altıokka-Uzun, G.; Tüzün, E.; Ekizoğlu, E.; Ulusoy, C.; Yentür, S.; Kürtüncü, M.; Saruhan-Direskeneli, G.; Baykan, B. Oligoclonal bands and increased cytokine levels in idiopathic intracranial hypertension. *Cephalalgia* **2015**, *35*, 1153–1161. [CrossRef]
17. Genizi, J.; Lahat, E.; Zelnik, N.; Mahajnah, M.; Ravid, S.; Shahar, E. Childhood-onset idiopathic intracranial hypertension: Relation of sex and obesity. *Pediatr. Neurol.* **2007**, *36*, 247–249. [CrossRef]
18. Cohen, R.; Mahajnah, M.; Shlonsky, Y.; Golan-Shany, O.; Romem, A.; Halevy, A.; Natan, K.; Genizi, J. Prospective, cross-sectional study finds no common viruses in cerebrospinal fluid of children with pseudotumor cerebri. *Brain Sci.* **2023**, *13*, 361. [CrossRef]
19. Park, G.; Fleifel, M.; Kesserwani, H.N. Pseudotumor cerebri secondary to jugular bulb thrombosis: A case report and a review of the diagnostic steps. *Cureus* **2022**, *14*, e27557. [CrossRef]

20. Kerty, E.; Heuser, K.; Indahl, U.G.; Berg, P.R.; Nakken, S.; Lien, S.; Omholt, S.W.; Ottersen, O.P.; Nagelhus, E.A. Is the brain water channel aquaporin-4 a pathogenetic factor in idiopathic intracranial hypertension? Results from a combined clinical and genetic study in a Norwegian cohort. *Acta Ophthalmol.* **2013**, *91*, 88–91. [CrossRef]
21. Lenck, S.; Radovanovic, I.; Nicholson, P.; Hodaie, M.; Krings, T.; Mendes-Pereira, V. Idiopathic intracranial hypertension: The veno glymphatic connections. *Neurology* **2018**, *91*, 515–522. [CrossRef] [PubMed]

children

MDPI

Communication

Neuromodulation in Pediatric Migraine Using Repetitive Neuromuscular Magnetic Stimulation: A Feasibility Study

Corinna Börner-Schröder [1,2,3,4,†], Magdalena Lang [1,2,†], Giada Urban [1,2], Erik Zaidenstadt [1,2], Jacob Staisch [1,2], Ari Hauser [1,2], Iris Hannibal [1,2], Kristina Huß [2], Birgit Klose [1,2], Matthias F. Lechner [1,2], Nico Sollmann [3,4,5], Mirjam N. Landgraf [1,2], Florian Heinen [1,2] and Michaela V. Bonfert [1,2,*]

1 Division of Pediatric Neurology and Developmental Medicine, Department of Pediatrics, Dr. Von Hauner Children's Hospital, LMU University Hospital, LMU Munich, 80337 Munich, Germany; corinna.boerner@med.lmu.de (C.B.-S.); iris.hannibal@med.lmu.de (I.H.); mirjam.landgraf@med.lmu.de (M.N.L.); florian.heinen@med.lmu.de (F.H.)

2 LMU Center for Children with Medical Complexity-iSPZ Hauner, LMU University Hospital, LMU Munich, 80337 Munich, Germany

3 Department of Diagnostic and Interventional Neuroradiology, School of Medicine, Klinikum Rechts der Isar, Technical University of Munich, Ismaninger Str. 22, 81675 Munich, Germany; nico.sollmann@tum.de

4 TUM-Neuroimaging Center, Klinikum Rechts der Isar, Technical University of Munich, 81675 Munich, Germany

5 Department of Diagnostic and Interventional Radiology, University Hospital Ulm, Albert-Einstein-Allee 23, 89081 Ulm, Germany

* Correspondence: michaela.bonfert@med.lmu.de; Tel.: +49-89-4400-55137; Fax: +49-89-4400-55166

† These authors were equally responsible for the work described in this paper.

Abstract: Migraine has a relevant impact on pediatric health. Non-pharmacological modalities for its management are urgently needed. This study assessed the safety, feasibility, acceptance, and efficacy of repetitive neuromuscular magnetic stimulation (rNMS) in pediatric migraine. A total of 13 patients with migraine, $\geq$6 headache days during baseline, and $\geq$1 myofascial trigger point in the upper trapezius muscles (UTM) received six rNMS sessions within 3 weeks. Headache frequency, intensity, and medication intake were monitored using headache calendars; headache-related impairment and quality of life were measured using PedMIDAS and KINDL questionnaires. Muscular involvement was assessed using pressure pain thresholds (PPT). Adherence yielded 100%. In 82% of all rNMS sessions, no side effects occurred. All participants would recommend rNMS and would repeat it. Headache frequency, medication intake, and PedMIDAS scores decreased from baseline to follow-up (FU), trending towards statistical significance ($p = 0.089$; $p = 0.081$, $p = 0.055$). A total of 7 patients were classified as responders, with a $\geq$25% relative reduction in headache frequency. PPT above the UTM significantly increased from pre- to post-assessment, which sustained until FU ($p = 0.015$ and 0.026, respectively). rNMS was safe, feasible, well-accepted, and beneficial on the muscular level. The potential to reduce headache-related symptoms together with PPT changes of the targeted UTM may underscore the interplay of peripheral and central mechanisms conceptualized within the trigemino-cervical complex.

Keywords: primary headache; responder rate; neurostimulation; pain pressure threshold; myofascial trigger point

1. Introduction

Migraine was one of the most prevalent neurological disorders worldwide in 2019 [1]. In children and adolescents, headache disorders are common and frequently associated with a high burden of disease as well [2–4]. Its negative impact on a child's quality of life, participation in school, sports or leisure time activities, and family life is very high [5,6]. Currently, a multi-modal interdisciplinary approach combining education, lifestyle management, behavioral therapy, and physiotherapy is recommended for children and adolescents affected by migraine [7–13]. Efficient pharmacological treatments for acute migraine attacks are available, whereas pharmaco-prophylaxis plays a secondary role in pediatric patients due to low evidence levels, oftentimes insufficient efficacy, and the risk of side effects [5,14–16]. Whether CGRP antibodies could represent an effective option in the future is currently being evaluated in a randomized clinical trial (https://clinicaltrials.gov/study/NCT03832998 accessed on 20 October 2023). However, data have not yet been published and will only refer to patients affected by chronic migraine. Hence, there is an increasing demand to develop non-pharmacological, non-invasive options as an addition to the contemporary multi-modal approach to pediatric migraine.

Concerning migraine pathophysiology, the trigemino-cervical complex (TCC) plays a major role [17–19], which describes the convergence of central and peripheral mechanisms of pain perception, processing, perpetuation, and sensitization [17]. Within this concept, reports of neck pain as well as findings during manual palpation of the neck and upper trapezius muscles (UTMs, e.g., myofascial trigger points (mTrP) [20–30]) can be interpreted as evidence for muscular involvement in patients with migraine [31,32].

The application of repetitive neuromuscular magnetic stimulation (rNMS) targeting the UTMs has been reported to be a safe and well-tolerated treatment option in adults affected by migraine, with encouraging results regarding the decrease in muscular hyperalgesia and headache symptoms [33–35]. Similar effects were described in an observational analysis among children and adolescents with headache disorders receiving rNMS in a tertiary outpatient headache center [36,37]. Through painless personalized electromagnetic induction, rNMS provokes an electric current in the stimulated body region [38]. This depolarizes motor and afferent nerves causing, among other effects, the muscle to contract. The resulting increased proprioceptive inflow to the central nervous system is hypothesized to modulate sensorimotor integration and pain processing pathways [15,38–42].

This study was designed to investigate the feasibility of the rNMS intervention in a cohort of children and adolescents affected by migraine by assessing the adherence to, safety of, and satisfaction with the treatment in a prospective design for the first time. In addition, the following clinical endpoints were preliminarily evaluated: changes in headache-related symptoms, including the burden of migraine and in quality of life, as well as the immediate local muscular effects of rNMS in terms of changes in pressure pain thresholds (PPT) above the UTMs.

2. Materials and Methods

2.1. Ethics and Study Enrollment

This study was approved by the institutional review board (vote 20-194) and registered in the German Clinical Trials Register (DRKS00022141). It was conducted in accordance with the Declaration of Helsinki. Written informed consent was obtained from all participants and their legal guardians.

2.2. Subjects

Participants were recruited via the outpatient headache center of our university's children's hospital. Inclusion criteria were (1) age 6 to 17 years, (2) a diagnosis of migraine according to the International Classification of Headache Disorders (ICHD 3rd edition) [43], (3) at least six headache days within a 90-day baseline assessment period, and (4) at least one mTrP in one of the UTMs. Regarding mTrP identification, the three standard criteria defining mTrP were carefully checked: (1) a palpable taut band with (2) hypersensitive spots and (3) a referred sensation/pain during manual palpation [22,44]. Exclusion criteria were (1) a diagnosis of familial hemiplegic migraine, (2) any pharmacological migraine prophylaxis except magnesium, (3) any other neurological/psychiatric disorders besides headaches, (4) any serious disease, and (5) contraindications for magnetic stimulation. As mixed-type headache (coexistence of migraine and TTH) is common in children and adolescents, a TTH component was not an exclusion criterion for study participation.

2.3. Prospective Study Design and rNMS Intervention

Enrollment took place consecutively between August 2020 and October 2021, with the last follow-up examination (FU) taking place in January 2022. During a 90-day baseline period, participants recorded the headache frequency and characteristics using a standardized headache calendar [45]. Subsequently, participants entered a 3-week intervention period consisting of 6 rNMS sessions targeting the UTM bilaterally with an eMFieldPro system (Zimmer Medizinsysteme GmbH, Neu-Ulm, Germany, CE Nr 0123). This study used the rNMS method described in the study of Staisch et al. (2022) and may partly reproduce the wording [36] (15 min, 20 Hz, 7 s ON time, 10 s OFF time; Figure 1). After the intervention, a 90-day FU period took place during in which subjects continued using their headache calendar.

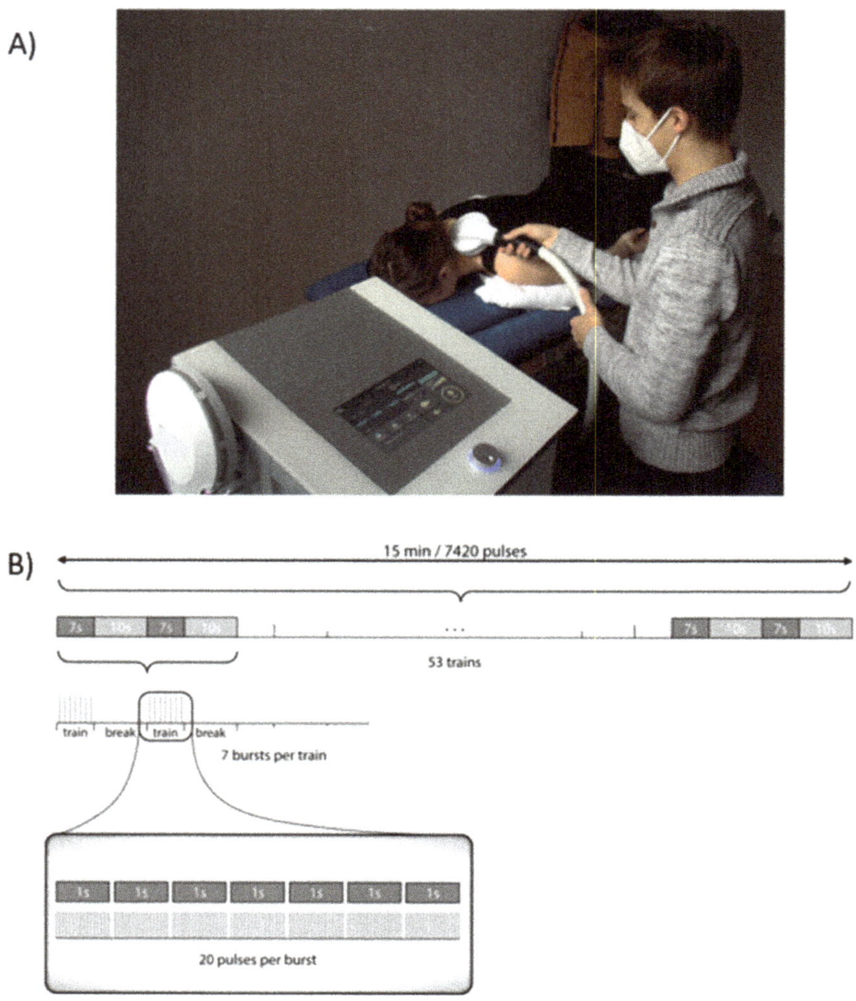

Figure 1. Clinical setup of rNMS treatment. (**A**) rNMS setting and coil positioning. (**B**) Stimulation protocol used for the rNMS treatments. Since 53 trains could not be visualized individually, which is why the repetition of trains is marked with [. . .]. Abbreviation: rNMS = repetitive neuromuscular magnetic stimulation.

2.4. Outcome Measures

This study used similar assessments as described in the study of Staisch et al. (2022) [36] and Börner et al. (2022) [37] and may partly reproduce the wording. Adherence: Adherence was defined as completing at least 5 of the 6 sessions of the rNMS intervention. If sessions were canceled, the reasons were asked for. Safety: A customized standardized questionnaire was used to assess any adverse events (AE) during or after stimulation. Satisfaction: After the intervention, patients and caregivers gave feedback on whether they would like to repeat or recommend rNMS using a customized standardized questionnaire. Clinical outcomes: During the whole course of the study, patients monitored headache symptoms using the headache calendar of the German Migraine and Headache Society [45]. Before the intervention and at FU 90 days after the intervention, headache-related impairment and quality of life were evaluated using the Pediatric Migraine Disability Assessment (PedMIDAS) [46] and a German generic quality of life instrument for patients and caregivers (KINDL questionnaire) [47]. Concurrently, subjects were asked to report life events having occurred during study participation. To identify mTrP in the UTM, a certified physiotherapist examined all participants using manual palpation at the time of screening, before and after the intervention, as well as during the FU exam 90 days after the intervention. In addition to mTrP assessments, reference points were defined as 1/3 and 2/3 of the distance from the vertebra C7 to the acromion above the left and right UTM to allow the investigation of changes in the whole musculature. Before and after each rNMS session as well as at FU examination 90 days after the intervention, PPT above each mTrP and all reference points were determined using algometry (Wagner Instrument, Greenwich, CT, USA). Measurements were performed three times per point.

2.5. Data Management

Data were pseudonymized and entered into Microsoft Excel data sheets (Microsoft Office Professional Plus 2016, Microsoft, Redmond, WA, USA). At least two independent analysts checked the data for plausibility. Based on the headache calendars covering 90 days, mean headache frequency, duration, and intensity were reported as headache days per month, hours, and with a 10-point visual analogue scale (VAS) (0 no pain, 10 extreme pain). A headache day was defined as a day with a headache lasting for at least two hours or shorter if headache specific medication was taken (according to the ICHD-3 [43]). Two patients documented the headache intensity on an alternative VAS scale (smaller range) and were therefore excluded from the headache intensity analysis. Two patients noted headache episodes consecutively without the use of the headache calendar template or exact dates, which is why they had to be excluded from the analysis separately comparing headache frequency in the first month, second months, and third months after rNMS treatment as well as from headache intensity and medication intake analyses due to missing information. PedMIDAS scores were available for 12 patients, since 1 patient was at preschool age and therefore not able to complete the PedMIDAS questionnaire as it is partly based on the child's participation in school. PedMIDAS scores can be categorized as follows: score of 0 to 10: little to none impairment, score of 11 to 30: mild impairment, score of 31 to 50: moderate impairment, and score >50: severe impairment [46]. The maximum pressure of the algometer was 10 kg/cm^2. If no pain was indicated when reaching 10 kg/cm^2, this pressure was defined as the PPT [48]. Based on the relative headache frequency reduction from baseline to FU, patients were assigned to one of four responder rate groups ($\geq$75%; $\geq$50%, $\geq$25%, <25%) [49]. The FU data regarding PPT were available for 12 patients as one FU examination was only possible via telephone.

2.6. Statistics

As this is the first prospective clinical study to deliver rNMS to a pediatric cohort affected by migraine, the study was primarily designed to assess its feasibility in this age group reflected by adherence to the intervention. As the primary endpoint, the adherence rate was calculated as the percentage of participants who did not discontinue the intervention. A threshold of completing at least 5 of the 6 per protocol sessions was defined as fulfilling adherence to the intervention. Assuming that 90% of participants would adhere to the intervention, a sample size of $n = 12$ to $n = 15$ participants was intended to treat based on the expected confidence intervals. For the additional qualitative feasibility endpoints, a sample size estimation was not reasonable. By the time the study had been designed, not any pediatric data for the application of rNMS in migraine were available to base a power analysis with regard to the clinical endpoints on.

All statistical analyses were performed using SPSS (version 26/27; IBM SPSS Statistics for Windows, Armonk, NY, USA). The statistical significance level was set to $\alpha = 0.05$ for all tests. Adherence rate was defined as the percentage of completed rNMS sessions. Absolute/relative frequencies, means, standard deviations, medians, and ranges were calculated for characteristics, side effects, and the intervention feedback.

Normality of headache variables, questionnaire scores, and PPT were analyzed using Shapiro–Wilk tests. Differences in headache frequency, headache intensity, frequency of days with medication intake, and the KINDL scores of caregivers from baseline to FU were evaluated using paired t-tests. Differences in headache duration, PedMIDAS scores, and KINDL scores of participants from baseline to FU were investigated using Wilcoxon signed-rank tests. Differences in monthly headache frequency were compared at 4 time points (baseline, one month, two months, and three months after rNMS treatment, respectively) using a repeated-measures ANOVA. The mean PPT above the left and right UTM was calculated as the average of the PPT above the lateral and medial reference points and the mTrP. Differences in PPT above the left and right UTM were assessed using repeated-measures ANOVAs for the following time points: (1) before the first rNMS session (pre), (2) before the last rNMS session (post), and (3) at FU. For ANOVAs, the Bonferroni correction was used for post hoc comparisons. In the case of a significant Mauchley's test of sphericity, the Greenhaus–Geisser correction was applied.

3. Results

3.1. Screening

A total of 248 patients treated at the outpatient headache center during the enrollment period were screened for eligibility, of whom 20 patients fulfilled all inclusion criteria (8.1%) and completed the baseline period. A total of 6 patients (2.4%) were excluded after the 90-day baseline period due to (1) less than six headache days within the baseline period ($n = 3$), (2) absence of mTrP in the UTM during manual palpation at the end of baseline ($n = 2$), and denial to participate in the intervention period ($n = 1$). One patient was excluded from analysis due to incongruence of the clinical diagnosis and the headache symptoms recorded by the headache calendar ($n = 1$). (Figure 2 and Supplementary Table S1).

3.2. Subject Characteristics

A total of 13 patients aged 12.2 ± 3.5 years (range: 6–17 years; 92.3% female) were enrolled in the study (Table 1 and Supplementary Table S2). A total of 3 patients were diagnosed with migraine with aura, of whom 2 patients additionally experienced tension type headache (TTH) characteristics. The remaining 10 patients were diagnosed with migraine without aura, with 5 patients also affected by TTH. The baseline mean headache frequency was 9.43 ± 5.86 headache days per month, with a median of 9.0 and an IQR 4.50–13.17 headache days per month. A total of 7 patients were experiencing neck pain at baseline; 6 patients received physiotherapy during baseline, 2 patients continued, and 1 patient started physiotherapy during the intervention period. All patients took acute medication: most patients used cyclooxygenase inhibitors ($n = 10$ ibuprofen, $n = 3$ naproxen, $n = 2$ acetylsalicylic acid); also triptans ($n = 4$) and paracetamol ($n = 2$) were prescribed. No patient took any preventive migraine medication, except magnesium ($n = 9$). Detailed subject and baseline characteristics are listed in Table 1.

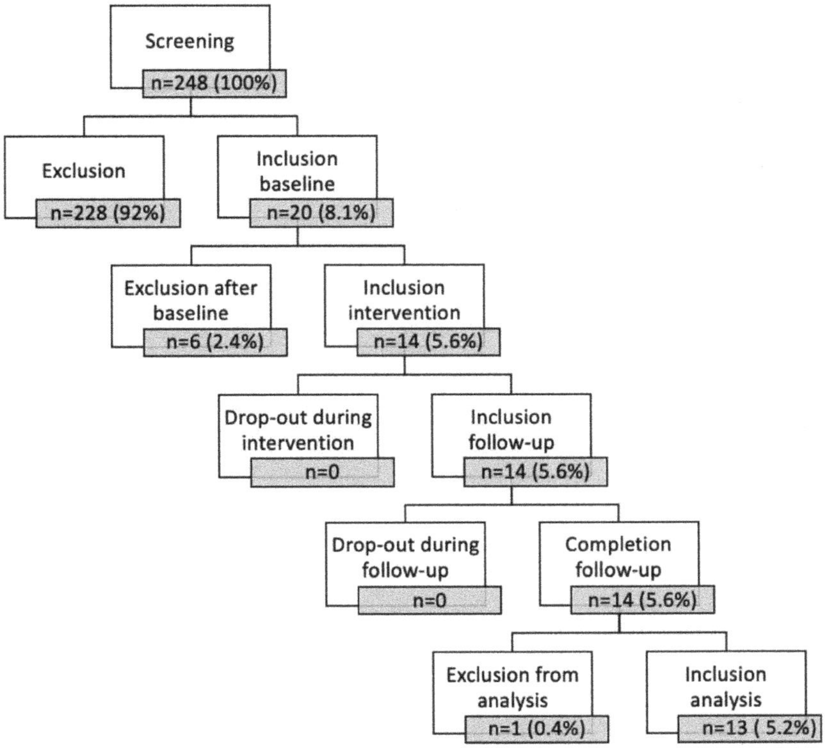

Figure 2. Screening scheme for study inclusion.

3.3. Treatment Characteristics

rNMS was performed with a mean stimulation intensity of 31.8 ± 12.3% of the maximum stimulator output on the left side and at 32.0 ± 11.6% of the maximum stimulator output on the right side.

3.4. Adherence

No dropouts were recorded. All participants completed all six rNMS sessions (adherence rate: 100%). Nine patients completed all sessions within a 3-week interval. For four patients, altogether eight sessions needed to be differently scheduled due to (1) acute illness of the patient (n = 2, 25%), (2) time constraints by the family (n = 1, 12.5%), (3) resource constraints by the outpatient clinic (n = 2, 25%), (4) absence without excuse (n = 2, 25%), and (5) accident due to weather conditions (n = 1, 12.5%) ending up in an intervention period of four to five weeks.

3.5. Safety

AEs were evaluated for 78 rNMS sessions. In 64 sessions (82.1%), no AEs were reported. A total of 16 side effects were reported for the remaining 14 rNMS sessions (17.9%) (Table 2). No AE led to discontinuation of the intervention.

Table 1. Characteristics of study participants (n = 13).

Characteristics		n (%)	Median (Range)
Age		-	12 (6–17)
Sex	Female	12 (92.3%)	-
Handedness	Right	10 (76.9%)	-
Headache Diagnosis			
Migraine with aura		1 (7.7%)	-
Migraine without aura		5 (38.5%)	-
Migraine with aura + TTH		2 (15.4%)	-
Migraine without aura + TTH		5 (38.5%)	-
Age at headache onset (years)		-	9 (2–15)
Time since headache onset (years)		-	3 (2–13)
Family history for migraine	Yes	3 (23.1%)	-
No		9 (69.2%)	-
Not known		1 (7.7%)	-
Neck pain at baseline	Yes	7 (53.8%)	-
No		6 (46.6%)	-
mTrP localization at baseline	Unilateral	5 (38.5%)	-
	Bilateral	8 (61.5%)	-
	Left	10 (45.5%)	-
Right		12 (54.5%)	-
mTrP entity at baseline	Latent	15 (68.2%)	-
Active		7 (31.8%)	-
Physiotherapy	During baseline	6 (46.2%)	-
During intervention		3 (23.1%)	-

Abbreviations: TTH = tension type headache, mTrP = myofascial trigger point.

Table 2. Adverse events (AEs) documented within n = 78 rNMS sessions.

AE (n = 91)	n (%)	Serious/Severe	Unexpected	Related
No side effects	64 (82.1%)			
Side effects	16 in 14 sessions (17.9%)			
During stimulation				
Trembling (arm/hand)	5 (6.4%)			X
Heaviness (at stimulation site)	2 (2.6%)			X
Tingling (at stimulation site)	1 (1.3%)			X
Arm pain	1 (1.3%)			X
Tension in shoulder-neck region (hand)	1 (1.3%)			X
In-between stimulations				
Headache	5 (6.4%)			X
Sore muscles	1 (1.3%)			X
Life events				
Suicide of school colleague	1 (7.7%)	X	X	
Health-related absence of caregiver [a]	1 (7.7%)			
Accident on ice	1 (7.7%)		X	

[a] For this variable, none of the criteria (serious/severe, unexpected, related) applied; they might have influenced the perception of headaches. Abbreviation: AE = adverse event.

3.6. Satisfaction

After the intervention, 13 subjects (100%) wanted to repeat rNMS and recommend it to other patients. A total of 13 caregivers (100%) would recommend rNMS to other children with migraine, and 10 caregivers (76.9%) would repeat the intervention. The reason why 3 caregivers did not indicate to repeat the treatment was that they themselves did not perceive a sufficient improvement in their child's treated headache.

3.7. Headache Characteristics

Headache frequency numerically decreased from 9.43 ± 5.86 days per month during the baseline period by 2.53 days per month to 6.90 ± 4.53 days per month during the FU period. This reduction did not reach statistical significance (t = −1.848, p = 0.089, Table 3). Although the numerical drop of the mean monthly headache frequency was pronounced in the first (6.27 ± 4.52 days/month) and second month (6.45 ± 7.12 days/month) compared to the third month (9.00 ± 6.65 days/month) after the intervention, no statistically significant change was reached at any of these timepoints compared to the mean baseline headache frequency (p = 0.204, F = 1.76; Supplementary Table S3).

Table 3. Change in headache characteristics, PedMIDAS scores, and KINDL scores from baseline to FU.

Headache Characteristics	Pre		FU		Test Values		95% CI of Mean Difference
	Mean (SD)	Median (IQR)	Mean (SD)	Median (IQR)	t/Z	p	
Headache frequency	9.43 (5.86)	9.00 (4.50–13.17)	6.90 (4.53)	5.60 (3.00–10.67)	t = 1.848	0.089	−0.45–5.52
Headache intensity	5.50 (0.97)	5.21 (4.75–6.73)	6.27 (1.47)	6.53 (4.24–7.09)	t = −1.68	0.142	−1.86–0.31
Headache duration	6.27 (4.82)	5.03 (3.56–7.35)	6.50 (4.70)	4.45 (2.59–9.41)	Z = −0.89	0.929	-
Medication frequency	4.42 (2.58)	4.33 (2.67–5.33)	2.73 (2.10)	2.00 (0.75–4.66)	t = 1.94	0.081	−0.25–3.65
PedMIDAS	35.00 (23.84)	24.00 (21.00–51.00)	20.67 (16.83)	16.00 (7.75–30.75)	Z = −1.92	0.055	-
KINDL Child	65.23 (19.02)	69.50 (46.13–82.75)	67.08 (18.04)	74.00 (58.38–79.25)	Z = −0.420	0.675	-
KINDL Caregiver	67.27 (11.99)	68.75 (58.38–77.63)	69.44 (9.64)	70.75 (61.50–78.75)	t = −1.038	0.320	−6.74–2.39

Comparisons were made using paired-samples t-tests or Wilcoxon signed-rank tests depending on normality. Abbreviations: pre = before the rNMS intervention, FU = follow-up, SD = standard deviation, IQR = interquartile range, CI = confidence interval, KINDL = Revidierter Fragebogen für KINDer und Jugendliche zur Erfassung der gesundheitsbezogenen Lebensqualität, PedMIDAS = Pediatric Migraine Disability Assessment.

Congruently, we registered a statistically non-significant reduction in medication frequency from 4.42 ± 2.58 days per month at baseline to 2.73 ± 2.10 days per month at FU (t = 1.94, p = 0.081) resulting in a mean reduction of 1.7 days per month. Headache intensity and duration did not relevantly change from baseline to FU.

Seven patients were classified as responders showing a relative reduction in headache frequency of ≥25%. Of these seven patients, headache frequency decreased ≥50% in three patients, of which two patients showed a reduction of ≥75%.

3.8. Headache-Related Disability

When comparing PedMIDAS scores at the group-level before intervention (35.00 ± 23.84) and at FU (20.67 ± 16.83), a transition from an average moderate to mild disability was observed (Z = −1.92, p = 0.055, Table 3). On the individual level, at baseline, "severe" disability was experienced by three patients, "moderate" disability by one patient, and "mild" disability by eight patients; no patient was categorized as "little to not" disabled (Figure 3). At FU, one patient was categorized as "severely", two patients as "moderately", six patients as "mildly", and three patients as "little to not" disabled. Two patients transitioned to a more severe category, whereas five patients turned to a less severe category, with one patient even dropping from "severe" to "little to none" disability. Five patients remained in their categories. Individual changes from baseline to FU in PedMIDAS scores, monthly headache frequency, intensity, and medication intake are depicted in Supplementary Table S4. No significant change in health-related quality of life was detected, neither in the total score of the KINDL questionnaire answered by the patient (baseline = 65.23 ± 19.02, FU = 67.08 ± 18.04, p = 0.675), nor in the questionnaire answered by the caregiver (baseline = 67.27 ± 11.99, FU = 69.44 ± 9.64, p = 0.320).

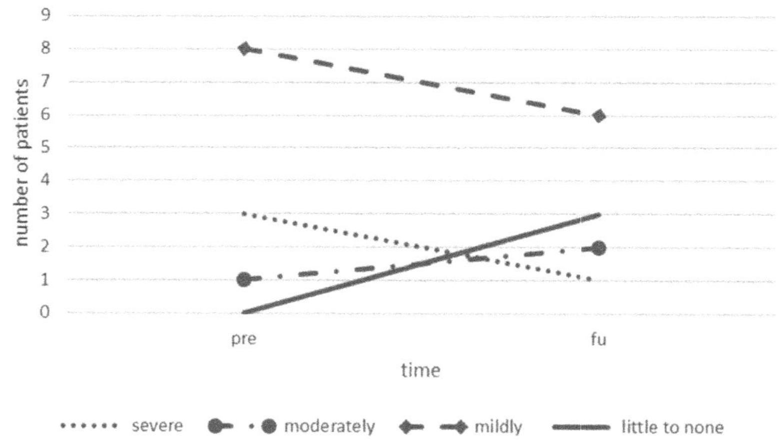

Figure 3. Comparison of PedMIDAS categories before and after rNMS treatment. Abbreviations: rNMS = repetitive neuromuscular magnetic stimulation, pre = before treatment, post = after treatment, PedMIDAS = Pediatric Migraine Disability Assessment.

3.9. *Muscular Effects*

Mean PPT measured above the left and right UTM significantly increased over time (left UTM: $p = 0.016$, right UTM: $p = 0.037$, Table 4 and Figure 4). Single comparisons of PPT above each assessed point (left lateral, left medial, left mTrP, right lateral, right medial, right mTrP) before and after the rNMS treatment are given in Supplementary Table S5.

Table 4. PPT comparison above the left and right UTM prior the first rNMS session (pre), prior the last rNMS session (post), and at the 3-month FU examination.

	Test Values			Mean_Pre (SD)	Mean_Post (SD)	Mean_FU (SD)	Post Hoc Test
	F	*p*	η^2				*p*
Left UTM	6.46	0.016 *	0.564	1.99 (0.77)	3.02 (1.61)	2.84 (1.13)	
Pre-post							0.097
Pre-FU							0.015 *
Post-FU							1.000
Right UTM	4.67	0.037 *	0.483	2.04 (0.67)	3.00 (1.55)	2.70 (1.00)	
Pre-post							0.126
Pre-FU							0.026 *
Post-FU							1.000

PPT comparisons above the left and right UTM using repeated-measures ANOVAs. Post hoc comparisons were performed with Bonferroni correction. Significant differences at $\alpha = 0.05$ are marked with an asterisk (*). Abbreviations: PPT = pressure pain threshold, UTM = upper trapezius muscle, FU = follow-up, pre = prior the first rNMS session, post = prior the last rNMS session, SD = standard deviation.

Of the seven patients with bilateral mTrP at baseline, one patient had only one unilateral mTrP at FU while the remaining six patients were still diagnosed with bilateral mTrP. Of five patients with unilateral mTrP at baseline (left n = one patient, right n = four patients), three patients had no mTrP at FU, while mTrP could be detected uni- and bilaterally in one patient, respectively.

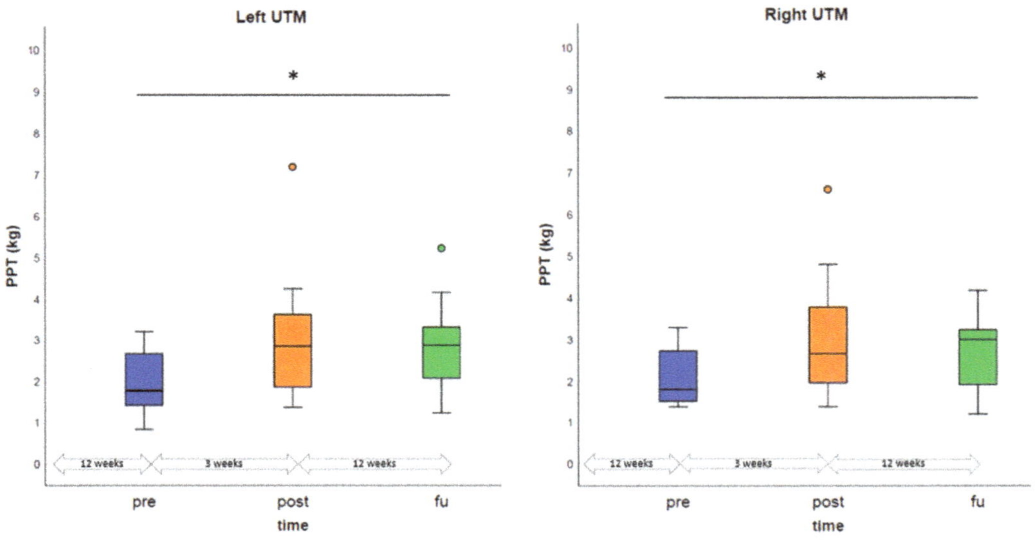

Figure 4. Comparison of PPT prior the first rNMS session, prior the last rNMS session, and at the 3-month FU examination. PPT above the left and right UTM were calculated based on the average of PPT above the lateral and medial reference points as well as the mTrP. Boxplots display the median PPT as well as the IQR. Significant differences are marked with an asterisk (*). Abbreviations: PPT = pressure pain threshold, mTrP = myofascial trigger point, pre = prior to the first rNMS session, post = prior to the last rNMS session, FU = follow-up, IQR = interquartile range.

4. Discussion

This study investigated the feasibility of the rNMS intervention as a non-pharmacological, non-invasive treatment option in a group of children affected by episodic migraine with involvement of the neck muscles. Feasibility measures were the adherence to, safety of, and satisfaction with the treatment. These measures were for the first time assessed in a prospective open-label design in this age group. In addition, preliminary clinical effects of the intervention were prospectively studied for the first time, not only focusing on changes in headache-related and muscular symptoms but on burden of migraine and in quality of life, too.

In this cohort, rNMS was feasible, safe, and well-accepted (adherence rate of 100%; no adverse events in 82.1% of rNMS sessions; 100% of patients would repeat and recommend rNMS). These results are in line with the findings from an observational report of rNMS as treatment in children and adolescents with different types of headache disorders, as well as to the results of studies involving adult participants [34–36].

Regarding the effects on headache-related symptoms, the monthly headache frequency and medication intake numerically decreased after the intervention, albeit without statistical significance. Importantly, seven patients (54%) were qualified as responders by experiencing a relief of their headache frequency by at least 25% and one additional participant reported a reduction close to the responder threshold (23%). This trend is comparable to findings in a cohort of children and adolescents with different types of headache disorders receiving rNMS, in that headache frequency and intensity were significantly reduced after rNMS (reduction from 17.1 ± 11.4 to 10.9 ± 10.9 headache days/month [mean $\pm$ SD]) [36] and comparable responder rates were observed for the group of participants affected by primary headaches, including nine patients with mixed-type headache and two with migraine only (43% responders in terms of $\geq$25% reduction, 14% responders in terms of $\geq$75% reduction) [36,37]. Similar findings have also been reported in previous studies investigating rNMS in young adults with episodic migraine (reduction in headache frequency from 7.7 (5.7–12) to 5.3 (1.7–10.3) days/month [median (range)] and 7.7 ± 6.9 to 5.1 ± 4.8 days/month [mean ± SD]; reduction in medication intake from 4 (0–9.7) to 3 (0–9) days/month [median (range)] and 3.3 ± 2.8 to 2.8 ± 1.8 days/month [mean ± SD]) [33,35]. Moreover, a retrospective analysis of the pooled data of both studies showed similar developments, too (reduction in headache frequency from 8.17 ± 4.50 to 6.33 ± 4.38 days/month [mean ± SD], reduction in medication intake from 3.63 ± 2.58 to 3.10 ± 2.44 days/month [mean ± SD]) [50].

With regard to headache-related disability, a significant reduction in MIDAS scores was reported after rNMS in adults with episodic migraine in previous studies (MIDAS Score reduction from 26.33 ± 13.89 to 15.37 ± 12.30 [mean ± SD]) [50]. In congruence, in the current first ever report on the impact of rNMS to the burden of migraine, PedMIDAS scores decreased on average by 14.33 units from baseline to FU, which corresponds to a reduction of 40.9%. These results are clinically meaningful, considering the highly problematic consequences of school absenteeism, and avoidance of physical and everyday activities in childhood due to migraine symptoms. Thus, a decreased PedMIDAS score likely reflects increased participation after rNMS, representing an important criterion regarding the treatment of pediatric migraine. In our pediatric cohort, more patients were classified as being mildly to not at all disabled after the rNMS intervention. With regard to the KINDL scores, no changes in health-related quality of life were reported after rNMS, neither by patients nor by their caregivers. However, it should be noted that baseline KINDL scores (65.23 ± 19.02) were already almost at the same level as reference values of healthy children in the KIGGS study ("Studie zur Gesundheit von Kindern und Jugendlichen in Deutschland", performed by the Robert Koch-Institute; mean: 76.90; 95% confidence interval 76.70–77.10) [51] and BELLA study ("BEfragung zum seeLischen WohLbefinden und VerhAlten", submodule of the KIGGS study; 76.30 ± 10.10) [52]. Hence, ceiling effects may have hampered the detection of further improvement.

Regarding muscular effects, the current analysis demonstrated an increase in PPT from pre- to post-assessments above the UTM, reflecting a relief of muscular hypersensitivity. This effect lasted until the 3-month FU, implicating that a decrease in local muscular hypersensitivity induced by rNMS can be sustained for a certain period of time. Of importance, in contrast to the long-term muscular effects of rNMS portrayed in this study, the majority of studies evaluating the effects of neuromodulation methods only included acute short-time FU (e.g., FU period of 10 min) [53–60]. Our findings are congruent with previous investigations of rNMS in children [37] as well as in adults affected by headaches. Our results show an increase in PPT from pre- to post-assessment of 0.96 ± 0.42 kg/cm^2 for the right and 1.03 ± 0.42 kg/cm^2 for the left UTM, which is comparable to PPT increases reported in the adult studies (right UTM: 0.4 (−1.1–2.5) kg/cm^2 [median (range)] and 0.8 kg/cm^2 [mean, SD for difference not given]; left UTM: 0.6 (−0.5–2.6) kg/cm^2 [median (range)] and 0.6 kg/cm^2 [mean, SD for difference not given]) [34,35]. PPT after rNMS measured above the UTM increased to a level of PPT measured in pediatric patients with chronic pain above the non-pain control sites and in a healthy reference population [61]. In addition, PPT above the UTM prior to rNMS were comparable or lower than PPT measured in adult migraine patients. PPT after rNMS were similar or even higher than PPT of healthy controls [62,63]. Together, this suggests an even more pronounced muscular hypersensitivity in pediatric patients than in healthy adults, which can potentially be reset to a level of healthy controls by rNMS targeting the UTM as a muscle considered part of the TCC. This may be interpreted as a sign of network reorganization via the TTC, eventually including the desensitization of the hypersensitive trigeminal nucleus caudalis [64].

Regarding the aspect of neuroinflammation in migraine pathogenesis, magnetic resonance imaging (MRI) studies suggest neuroinflammatory mechanisms on the muscular level [65,66], in addition to the well-described CGRP-related (Calcitonin Gene-Related Peptide) alterations on the leptomeningeal vascular level [67,68]. The relief of muscular symptoms (e.g., increased PPT, decreased number of mTrP) by rNMS points at a possible relief from muscular neuroinflammation. In addition to the beneficial clinical effects, the important interplay of the peripheral and central networks is emphasized, once more. This context might call for further in-depth investigations of alterations of muscles involved in migraine pathogenesis via the TCC, i.e., by advanced imaging on behalf of T2 mapping and other advances MRI-based techniques [65,66].

Neurostimulation as acute or prophylactic migraine treatment is quite a novel approach; thus, the number of studies is still limited to date and no data exist for the pediatric population for the majority of modalities [7,69]. For the acute migraine treatment and migraine prophylaxis, the following approaches have been investigated: transcranial magnetic stimulation [70], transcranial direct current stimulation [71], transcutaneous occipital nerve stimulation [53,72], transcutaneous supraorbital nerve stimulation [54,73], transcutaneous vagus nerve stimulation [74,75], and remote electrical neuromodulation [60]. In comparison to the abovementioned techniques, rNMS specifically targets the muscle and could treat the muscular level in addition to central effectors—including in children and adolescents. Specifically, it has several aspects that might facilitate its use in the pediatric setting, including in particular a painless application. Therefore, rNMS may be better accepted by patients, which is an important factor in the pediatric field [36,69,76]. Regarding the association of migraine, neck pain, and muscular hypersensitivity, rNMS is unique in targeting both the muscular and the central pathophysiological mechanisms conceptualized within the framework of the TCC [17,19], which is achieved via a single "from bottom-up" approach [69]. Thus, rNMS may represent a valuable non-invasive, non-pharmacological component within the future treatment concepts for pediatric migraine. Against the background of these promising results in children, data from large-scale randomized controlled trials in adults are expected to pave the way for a widespread application of rNMS across all age groups (https://drks.de/search/de/trial/DRKS00024470 accessed on 20 October 2023).

As this study included a rather small cohort of 13 patients with migraine, findings are not generalizable to the whole population of pediatric patients affected by migraine. Despite the small cohort, the assumption that 90% of participants would adhere to the intervention led to a sample size calculation of $n = 12$ to $n = 15$ participants needing to be treated to reach reasonable confidence intervals (CI $\pm$ 15.2 to $\pm$ 16.9), which enhances the reliability of the effects despite the sample size limitation. Yet, given the strict in- and exclusion criteria, the data represent the feasibility and preliminary effects in a cohort of pediatric patients affected by migraine as clinically homogenously as possible. In particular, assuring a relatively high baseline frequency of headaches and the presence of muscular involvement through an expert manual palpation, together with the rule out of comorbidities like somatoform or psychiatric disorders, represent important quality criteria of the study. Another reason for limitations in the sample size had been the ongoing COVID-19 pandemic, that restricted outpatient contacts to a minimum. Given the age range of the study population, no conclusions regarding when to start a neurostimulation during the trajectory of migraine can be drawn. Headache documentation is especially challenging in children and adolescents, which should be considered when interpreting the reported results. Novel, digitalized kids-friendly applications are urgently needed to ensure a more feasible headache documentation in clinical practice and research. Regarding muscular effects, only one FU examination took place 90 days after the intervention. While numerically decreased headache frequency was pronounced during the first and second month after the intervention, no conclusions regarding trajectory or wear-off effects regarding the muscular symptoms can be made to date. Future studies should therefore consider implementing physiotherapeutic assessment at several time points during FU and may additionally implement objective point-of-care imaging measures to assess muscular changes (e.g., muscular ultrasound or infrared thermography). Furthermore, the lack of objective neurophysiological outcome measures (e.g., fMRI) limits the interpretability of the here-reported rNMS effects, and further studies including neurophysiological outcome measures are needed to underpin the pathophysiological hypothesis of the distinct mechanisms of action of rNMS in migraine. Concerning algometry, it should be noticed that measurements in young children (6–8 years) may not be as reliable as in adults or older children, which is due to difficulties in describing perceptions and a higher sensitivity to pain stimuli [63]. A setting effect may have affected the here-presented outcomes, especially since this effect might be higher in the pediatric population in general [5,11,77]. Furthermore, there may be an increased placebo response to interventions using a medical device compared to pharmacologic treatment modalities [77]. In addition, three psychosocial AEs were reported by three patients during the study period, which may have interfered with the effects reported here. Since the study was carried out during the COVID-19 pandemic, the closure of schools, sports clubs, and recreational facilities, social distancing, and the rapid change in legal restrictions may have affected the patients' daily routine, as well as overall quality of life and burden of headache. Since migraine is a very common disorder in pediatric age but nevertheless characterized as one of the most underfunded diseases [78,79], more sham-controlled studies investigating non-pharmacological, non-invasive treatment options for pediatric patients are urgently needed.

5. Conclusions

rNMS interventions were safe, feasible, and well-accepted by children and adolescents with migraine. Although statistically non-significant, the monthly headache frequency, medication intake, and—particularly important and reported for the first time in this context—PedMIDAS scores demonstrated a relevant decrease from baseline to FU on an individual basis. Together with the potential to reduce the symptoms on the muscular level, rNMS might become a valuable option introducing neuromodulation from bottom up to the multimodal armentarium for children with episodic migraine. Therefore, future controlled studies are highly needed to further assess the current beneficial findings and to elucidate the specific neurophysiological mechanisms of rNMS in peripheral and central processes of pain processing.

Supplementary Materials: The following supporting information can be downloaded at: https://www.mdpi.com/article/10.3390/children10111764/s1; Table S1: Screening. Screening and reasons of exclusion; Table S2: Participants' characteristics. More detailed characteristics of the study participants; Table S3: Changes in monthly headache frequency of $n = 11$ patients for the first month, second month, and third month after rNMS intervention compared to baseline; Table S4: Individual changes from baseline to FU in PedMIDAS scores, monthly headache frequency, headache intensity, and medication intake; Table S5: (A) Comparison of PPT before the first (pre1) and before the last treatment sessions (pre6). (B) Comparison of PPT after the first (post1) and after the last treatment sessions (post6).

Author Contributions: Conceptualization, N.S., M.N.L., F.H. and M.V.B.; data curation, C.B.-S., M.L., E.Z., J.S., A.H. and M.V.B.; formal analysis, C.B.-S., M.L. and M.V.B.; investigation, C.B.-S., M.L., E.Z., J.S., A.H., I.H., K.H., B.K., M.F.L. and M.V.B.; methodology, C.B.-S., M.L., G.U., N.S. and M.V.B.; project administration, C.B.-S., M.L. and M.V.B.; resources, M.N.L., F.H. and M.V.B.; supervision, N.S., M.N.L., F.H. and M.V.B.; validation, C.B.-S., M.L. and M.V.B.; visualization, C.B.-S., M.L., E.Z., J.S. and A.H.; writing—original draft, C.B.-S., M.L. and M.V.B.; writing—review and editing, C.B.-S., M.L., G.U., E.Z., J.S., A.H., I.H., K.H., B.K., M.F.L., N.S., M.N.L., F.H. and M.V.B. All authors have read and agreed to the published version of the manuscript.

Funding: This publication did not receive any specific grant from funding agencies in the public, commercial, or not-for-profit sectors.

Institutional Review Board Statement: The study was conducted in accordance with the Declaration of Helsinki, and approved by the Institutional Review Board of the LMU Munich (protocol code 20-194, 15 April 2020).

Informed Consent Statement: Informed consent was obtained from all subjects involved in the study.

Data Availability Statement: The data presented in this study are available on request from the corresponding author. The data are not publicly available due to the sensitive character of pediatric clinical data.

Conflicts of Interest: The Division of Pediatric Neurology and Developmental Medicine, Dr. von Hauner Children's Hospital, LMU Hospital, Munich Germany was provided by an emFieldPro magnetic stimulator by Zimmer MedizinSysteme GmbH (Neu-Ulm, Germany). N.S. received honoraria from Nexstim Plc (Helsinki, Finland). M.N.L. and F.H. received a grant "Innovationsfonds" of the joint federal committee of health insurance companies (GBA) for a nation-wide study on an early multimodal intervention program for children with migraine. No further conflicts of interest are reported. MVB's research concerning neuromodulation in migraine is supported by a scholarship of the Bavarian Gender Equality Grant of the Free State of Bavaria, Germany. MVB's research concerning pediatric mTBI is supported by the ZNS-Hannelore Kohl Stiftung. MVB's and NS' research on rNMS in adult migraine are supported by a research grant of the Deutsche Migräne- und Kopfschmerzgesellschaft (DMKG).

References

1. GBD 2019 Diseases and Injuries Collaborators. Global burden of 369 diseases and injuries in 204 countries and territories, 1990–2019: A systematic analysis for the Global Burden of Disease Study 2019. *Lancet* **2020**, *396*, 1204–1222. [CrossRef]
2. Albers, L.; Straube, A.; Landgraf, M.N.; Filippopulos, F.; Heinen, F.; von Kries, R. Migraine and tension type headache in adolescents at grammar school in Germany—Burden of disease and health care utilization. *J. Headache Pain* **2015**, *16*, 52. [CrossRef]
3. Albers, L.; von Kries, R.; Heinen, F.; Straube, A. Headache in School Children: Is the Prevalence Increasing? *Curr. Pain Headache Rep.* **2015**, *19*, 4. [CrossRef]
4. Abu-Arafeh, I.; Razak, S.; Sivaraman, B.; Graham, C. Prevalence of headache and migraine in children and adolescents: A systematic review of population-based studies. *Dev. Med. Child Neurol.* **2010**, *52*, 1088–1097. [CrossRef] [PubMed]
5. E Youssef, P.; Mack, K.J. Episodic and chronic migraine in children. *Dev. Med. Child Neurol.* **2020**, *62*, 34–41. [CrossRef] [PubMed]
6. Katsuki, M.; Matsumori, Y.; Kawahara, J.; Yamagishi, C.; Koh, A.; Kawamura, S.; Kashiwagi, K.; Kito, T.; Oguri, M.; Mizuno, S.; et al. School-based online survey on chronic headache, migraine, and medication-overuse headache prevalence among children and adolescents in Japanese one city—Itoigawa Benizuwaigani study. *Clin. Neurol. Neurosurg.* **2023**, *226*, 107610. [CrossRef]
7. Bonfert, M.V.; Börner, C.; Gerstl, L.; Hannibal, I.; Mathonia, N.; Huß, K.; Rahmsdorf, B.; Kainz, C.; Klose, B.; Koenig, H.; et al. Migraine in childhood and adolescence-neurostimulation as a future innovative approach in terms of a multimodal treatment regimen. *Bundesgesundheitsblatt Gesundheitsforschung Gesundheitsschutz* **2020**, *63*, 872–880. [CrossRef]
8. Orr, S.L.; Kabbouche, M.A.; O'brien, H.L.; Kacperski, J.; Powers, S.W.; Hershey, A.D. Paediatric migraine: Evidence-based management and future directions. *Nat. Rev. Neurol.* **2018**, *14*, 515–527. [CrossRef] [PubMed]
9. Landgraf, M.N.; Heinen, F.; Gerstl, L.; Kainz, C.; Ruscheweyh, R.; Straube, A.; Scheidt, J.; von Mutius, S.; Obermeier, V.; von Kries, R. Comparison of a pediatric practice-based therapy and an interdisciplinary ambulatory treatment in social pediatric centers for migraine in children: A nation-wide randomized-controlled trial in Germany: "Moma—Modules on migraine activity". *BMC Pediatr.* **2021**, *21*, 294. [CrossRef]
10. National Institute for Health and Care Excellence (NICE). *National Institute for Health and Care Excellence: Clinical Guidelines*; National Institute for Health and Care Excellence (NICE): London, UK, 2021.
11. Oskoui, M.; Pringsheim, T.; Billinghurst, L.; Potrebic, S.; Gersz, E.M.; Gloss, D.; Holler-Managan, Y.; Leininger, E.; Licking, N.; Mack, K.; et al. Practice guideline update summary: Pharmacologic treatment for pediatric migraine prevention: Report of the Guideline Development, Dissemination, and Implementation Subcommittee of the American Academy of Neurology and the American Headache Society. *Neurology* **2019**, *93*, 500–509. [CrossRef]
12. Oskoui, M.; Pringsheim, T.; Holler-Managan, Y.; Potrebic, S.; Billinghurst, L.; Gloss, D.; Hershey, A.D.; Licking, N.; Sowell, M.; Victorio, M.C.; et al. Practice guideline update summary: Acute treatment of migraine in children and adolescents: Report of the Guideline Development, Dissemination, and Implementation Subcommittee of the American Academy of Neurology and the American Headache Society. *Neurology* **2019**, *93*, 487–499. [CrossRef] [PubMed]
13. Straube, A.; Schroeder, A.S.; Reilich, P.; Ebinger, F.; Heinen, F.; Bonfert, M. Primary Headache in Children and Adolescents: Update on Pharmacotherapy of Migraine and Tension-Type Headache. *Neuropediatrics* **2013**, *44*, 3–19. [CrossRef] [PubMed]
14. Diener, H.-C.; Charles, A.; Goadsby, P.J.; Holle, D. New therapeutic approaches for the prevention and treatment of migraine. *Lancet Neurol.* **2015**, *14*, 1010–1022. [CrossRef] [PubMed]
15. Charles, A. The pathophysiology of migraine: Implications for clinical management. *Lancet Neurol.* **2018**, *17*, 174–182. [CrossRef] [PubMed]
16. Lewis, D.; Ashwal, S.; Hershey, A.; Hirtz, D.; Yonker, M.; Silberstein, S. Practice Parameter: Pharmacological treatment of migraine headache in children and adolescents: Report of the American Academy of Neurology Quality Standards Subcommittee and the Practice Committee of the Child Neurology Society. *Neurology* **2004**, *63*, 2215–2224. [CrossRef] [PubMed]
17. Bartsch, T.; Goadsby, P.J. The trigeminocervical complex and migraine: Current concepts and synthesis. *Curr. Pain Headache Rep.* **2003**, *7*, 371–376. [CrossRef]
18. Busch, V.; Frese, A.; Bartsch, T. The trigemino-cervical complex. Integration of peripheral and central pain mechanisms in primary headache syndromes. *Schmerz* **2004**, *18*, 404–410. [CrossRef]

19. Ashina, M.; Hansen, J.M.; Do, T.P.; Melo-Carrillo, A.; Burstein, R.; A Moskowitz, M. Migraine and the trigeminovascular system—40 years and counting. *Lancet Neurol.* **2019**, *18*, 795–804. [CrossRef]
20. Landgraf, M.; Ertl-Wagner, B.; Koerte, I.; Thienel, J.; Langhagen, T.; Straube, A.; von Kries, R.; Reilich, P.; Pomschar, A.; Heinen, F. Alterations in the trapezius muscle in young patients with migraine—A pilot case series with MRI. *Eur. J. Paediatr. Neurol.* **2015**, *19*, 372–376. [CrossRef]
21. Landgraf, M.N.; von Kries, R.; Heinen, F.; Langhagen, T.; Straube, A.; Albers, L. Self-reported neck and shoulder pain in adolescents is associated with episodic and chronic migraine. *Cephalalgia* **2016**, *36*, 807–811. [CrossRef]
22. Fernández-De-Las-Peñas, C.; Dommerholt, J. International Consensus on Diagnostic Criteria and Clinical Considerations of Myofascial Trigger Points: A Delphi Study. *Pain Med.* **2018**, *19*, 142–150. [CrossRef] [PubMed]
23. Fernández-De-Las-Peñas, C.; Madeleine, P.; Caminero, A.; Cuadrado, M.; Arendt-Nielsen, L.; Pareja, J. Generalized Neck-Shoulder Hyperalgesia in Chronic Tension-Type Headache and Unilateral Migraine Assessed by Pressure Pain Sensitivity Topographical Maps of the Trapezius Muscle. *Cephalalgia* **2010**, *30*, 77–86. [CrossRef] [PubMed]
24. Fernández-De-Las-Peñas, C. Myofascial Head Pain. *Curr. Pain Headache Rep.* **2015**, *19*, 28. [CrossRef]
25. Blaschek, A.; Decke, S.; Albers, L.; Schroeder, A.S.; Lehmann, S.; Straube, A.; Landgraf, M.N.; Heinen, F.; von Kries, R. Self-reported neck pain is associated with migraine but not with tension-type headache in adolescents. *Cephalalgia* **2014**, *34*, 895–903. [CrossRef] [PubMed]
26. Blaschek, A.; Milde-Busch, A.; Straube, A.; Schankin, C.; Langhagen, T.; Jahn, K.; Schröder, S.A.; Reiter, K.; von Kries, R.; Heinen, F. Self-reported muscle pain in adolescents with migraine and tension-type headache. *Cephalalgia* **2012**, *32*, 241–249. [CrossRef]
27. Luedtke, K.; Starke, W.; May, A. Musculoskeletal dysfunction in migraine patients. *Cephalalgia* **2018**, *38*, 865–875. [CrossRef]
28. Simons, D.G.; Travell, J.G.; Simons, L.S. *Travell & Simons' Myofascial Pain and Dysfunction: Upper Half of Body*; Williams & Wilkins: Philadelphia, PA, USA, 1999.
29. Ferracini, G.N.; Florencio, L.L.; Dach, F.; Grossi, D.B.; Palacios-Ceña, M.; Ordás-Bandera, C.; Chaves, T.C.; Speciali, J.G.; Fernández-De-Las-Peñas, C. Musculoskeletal disorders of the upper cervical spine in women with episodic or chronic migraine. *Eur. J. Phys. Rehabil. Med.* **2017**, *53*, 342–350. [CrossRef]
30. Ashina, S.; Bendtsen, L.; Lyngberg, A.C.; Lipton, R.B.; Hajiyeva, N.; Jensen, R. Prevalence of neck pain in migraine and tension-type headache: A population study. *Cephalalgia* **2015**, *35*, 211–219. [CrossRef]
31. Do, T.P.; Heldarskard, G.F.; Kolding, L.T.; Hvedstrup, J.; Schytz, H.W. Myofascial trigger points in migraine and tension-type headache. *J. Headache Pain* **2018**, *19*, 84. [CrossRef]
32. Giamberardino, M.A.; Tafuri, E.; Savini, A.; Fabrizio, A.; Affaitati, G.; Lerza, R.; Di Ianni, L.; Lapenna, D.; Mezzetti, A. Contribution of Myofascial Trigger Points to Migraine Symptoms. *J. Pain* **2007**, *8*, 869–878. [CrossRef]
33. Renner, T.; Sollmann, N.; Heinen, F.; Albers, L.; Trepte-Freisleder, F.; Klose, B.; König, H.; Krieg, S.M.; Bonfert, M.V.; Landgraf, M.N. Alleviation of migraine symptoms by application of repetitive peripheral magnetic stimulation to myofascial trigger points of neck and shoulder muscles—A randomized trial. *Sci. Rep.* **2020**, *10*, 5954. [CrossRef] [PubMed]
34. Renner, T.; Sollmann, N.; Trepte-Freisleder, F.; Albers, L.; Mathonia, N.M.; Bonfert, M.V.; König, H.; Klose, B.; Krieg, S.M.; Heinen, F.; et al. Repetitive Peripheral Magnetic Stimulation (rPMS) in Subjects With Migraine—Setup Presentation and Effects on Skeletal Musculature. *Front. Neurol.* **2019**, *10*, 738. [CrossRef] [PubMed]
35. Sollmann, N.; Trepte-Freisleder, F.; Albers, L.; Jung, N.H.; Mall, V.; Meyer, B.; Heinen, F.; Krieg, S.M.; Landgraf, M.N. Magnetic stimulation of the upper trapezius muscles in patients with migraine—A pilot study. *Eur. J. Paediatr. Neurol.* **2016**, *20*, 888–897. [CrossRef] [PubMed]
36. Staisch, J.; Börner, C.; Lang, M.; Hauser, A.; Hannibal, I.; Huß, K.; Klose, B.; Lechner, M.F.; Sollmann, N.; Heinen, F.; et al. Repetitive neuromuscular magnetic stimulation in children with headache. *Eur. J. Paediatr. Neurol.* **2022**, *39*, 40–48. [CrossRef]
37. Börner, C.; Staisch, J.; Lang, M.; Hauser, A.; Hannibal, I.; Huß, K.; Klose, B.; Lechner, M.F.; Sollmann, N.; Heinen, F.; et al. Repetitive Neuromuscular Magnetic Stimulation for Pediatric Headache Disorders: Muscular Effects and Factors Affecting Level of Response. *Brain Sci.* **2022**, *12*, 932. [CrossRef]
38. Smania, N.; Corato, E.; Fiaschi, A.; Pietropoli, P.; Aglioti, S.M.; Tinazzi, M. Repetitive magnetic stimulation A novel therapeutic approach for myofascial pain syndrome. *J. Neurol.* **2005**, *252*, 307–314. [CrossRef]
39. Pujol, J.; Pascual-Leone, A.; Dolz, C.; Delgado, E.; Dolz, J.L.; Aldomà, J. The effect of repetitive magnetic stimulation on localized musculoskeletal pain. *NeuroReport* **1998**, *9*, 1745–1748. [CrossRef]
40. Bartsch, T.; Goadsby, P.J. Central mechanisms of peripheral nerve stimulation in headache disorders. *Prog. Neurol. Surg.* **2011**, *24*, 16–26. [CrossRef]
41. Beaulieu, L.; Schneider, C. Effects of repetitive peripheral magnetic stimulation on normal or impaired motor control. A review. *Neurophysiol. Clin.* **2013**, *43*, 251–260. [CrossRef]
42. Beaulieu, L.-D.; Schneider, C. Repetitive peripheral magnetic stimulation to reduce pain or improve sensorimotor impairments: A literature review on parameters of application and afferents recruitment. *Neurophysiol. Clin.* **2015**, *45*, 223–237. [CrossRef]
43. Headache Classification Committee of the International Headache Society (IHS). The International Classification of Headache Disorders, 3rd edition (beta version). *Cephalalgia* **2013**, *33*, 629–808. [CrossRef] [PubMed]
44. Fernández-De-Las-Peñas, C.; Simons, D.G.; Cuadrado, M.L.; Pareja, J.A. The role of myofascial trigger points in musculoskeletal pain syndromes of the head and neck. *Curr. Pain Headache Rep.* **2007**, *11*, 365–372. [CrossRef] [PubMed]

45. Jensen, R.; Tassorelli, C.; Rossi, P.; Allena, M.; Osipova, V.; Steiner, T.; Sandrini, G.; Olesen, J.; Nappi, G.; Barrientos, N.; et al. A basic diagnostic headache diary (BDHD) is well accepted and useful in the diagnosis of headache. A multicentre European and Latin American study. *Cephalalgia* **2011**, *31*, 1549–1560. [CrossRef] [PubMed]
46. Hershey, A.D.; Powers, S.W.; Vockell, A.-L.B.; LeCates, S.; Kabbouche, M.; Maynard, M.K. PedMIDAS: Development of a questionnaire to assess disability of migraines in children. *Neurology* **2001**, *57*, 2034–2039. [CrossRef] [PubMed]
47. Ravens-Sieberer, U.; Bullinger, M. Assessing health-related quality of life in chronically ill children with the German KINDL: First psychometric and content analytical results. *Qual. Life Res.* **1998**, *7*, 399–407. [CrossRef]
48. Lacourt, T.E.; Houtveen, J.H.; van Doornen, L.J. Experimental pressure-pain assessments: Test-retest reliability, convergence and dimensionality. *Scand. J. Pain* **2012**, *3*, 31–37. [CrossRef]
49. Tassorelli, C.; Diener, H.-C.; Dodick, D.W.; Silberstein, S.D.; Lipton, R.B.; Ashina, M.; Becker, W.J.; Ferrari, M.D.; Goadsby, P.J.; Pozo-Rosich, P.; et al. Guidelines of the International Headache Society for controlled trials of preventive treatment of chronic migraine in adults. *Cephalalgia* **2018**, *38*, 815–832. [CrossRef]
50. Börner, C.; Renner, T.; Trepte-Freisleder, F.; Urban, G.; Schandelmaier, P.; Lang, M.; Lechner, M.F.; Koenig, H.; Klose, B.; Albers, L.; et al. Response Predictors of Repetitive Neuromuscular Magnetic Stimulation in the Preventive Treatment of Episodic Migraine. *Front. Neurol.* **2022**, *13*, 919623. [CrossRef]
51. Ravens-Sieberer, U.; Ellert, U.; Erhart, M. Health-related quality of life of children and adolescents in Germany. Norm data from the German Health Interview and Examination Survey (KiGGS). *Bundesgesundheitsblatt—Gesundheitsforschung—Gesundheitsschutz* **2007**, *50*, 810–818. [CrossRef]
52. Ravens-Sieberer, U.; Erhart, M.; Wille, N.; Bullinger, M.; The BELLA Study Group. Health-related quality of life in children and adolescents in Germany: Results of the BELLA study. *Eur. Child Adolesc. Psychiatry* **2008**, *17*, 148–156. [CrossRef]
53. Bono, F.; Salvino, D.; Mazza, M.R.; Curcio, M.; Trimboli, M.; Vescio, B.; Quattrone, A. The influence of ictal cutaneous allodynia on the response to occipital transcutaneous electrical stimulation in chronic migraine and chronic tension-type headache: A randomized, sham-controlled study. *Cephalalgia* **2015**, *35*, 389–398. [CrossRef] [PubMed]
54. Schoenen, J.; Vandersmissen, B.; Jeangette, S.; Herroelen, L.; Vandenheede, M.; Gérard, P.; Magis, D. Migraine prevention with a supraorbital transcutaneous stimulator: A randomized controlled trial. *Neurology* **2013**, *80*, 697–704. [CrossRef] [PubMed]
55. Chou, D.E.; Yugrakh, M.S.; Winegarner, D.; Rowe, V.; Kuruvilla, D.; Schoenen, J. Acute migraine therapy with external trigeminal neurostimulation (ACME): A randomized controlled trial. *Cephalalgia* **2019**, *39*, 3–14. [CrossRef]
56. Jiang, L.; Yuan, D.L.; Li, M.; Liu, C.; Liu, Q.; Zhang, Y.; Tan, G. Combination of flunarizine and transcutaneous supraorbital neurostimulation improves migraine prophylaxis. *Acta Neurol. Scand.* **2019**, *139*, 276–283. [CrossRef] [PubMed]
57. Hokenek, N.M.; Erdogan, M.O.; Hokenek, U.D.; Algin, A.; Tekyol, D.; Seyhan, A.U. Treatment of migraine attacks by transcutaneous electrical nerve stimulation in emergency department: A randomize controlled trial. *Am. J. Emerg. Med.* **2021**, *39*, 80–85. [CrossRef]
58. Straube, A.; Ellrich, J.; Eren, O.; Blum, B.; Ruscheweyh, R. Treatment of chronic migraine with transcutaneous stimulation of the auricular branch of the vagal nerve (auricular t-VNS): A randomized, monocentric clinical trial. *J. Headache Pain* **2015**, *16*, 543. [CrossRef]
59. Silberstein, S.D.; Calhoun, A.H.; Lipton, R.B.; Grosberg, B.M.; Cady, R.K.; Dorlas, S.; Simmons, K.A.; Mullin, C.; Liebler, E.J.; Goadsby, P.J.; et al. Chronic migraine headache prevention with noninvasive vagus nerve stimulation. *Neurology* **2016**, *87*, 529–538. [CrossRef]
60. Yarnitsky, D.; Dodick, D.W.; Grosberg, B.M.; Burstein, R.; Ironi, A.; Harris, D.; Lin, T.; Silberstein, S.D. Remote Electrical Neuromodulation (REN) Relieves Acute Migraine: A Randomized, Double-Blind, Placebo-Controlled, Multicenter Trial. *Headache J. Head Face Pain* **2019**, *59*, 1240–1252. [CrossRef]
61. Kersch, A.; Perera, P.; Mercado, M.; Gorrie, A.; Sainsbury, D.; McGrath, T.; Aouad, P.; Sarraf, S.; Jaaniste, T.; Champion, D. Somatosensory Testing in Pediatric Patients with Chronic Pain: An Exploration of Clinical Utility. *Children* **2020**, *7*, 275. [CrossRef]
62. Florencio, L.L.; Giantomassi, M.C.M.; Carvalho, G.F.; Gonçalves, M.C.; Dach, F.; Fernández-De-Las-Peñas, C.; Bevilaqua-Grossi, D. Generalized Pressure Pain Hypersensitivity in the Cervical Muscles in Women with Migraine. *Pain Med.* **2015**, *16*, 1629–1634. [CrossRef]
63. Blankenburg, M.; Boekens, H.; Hechler, T.; Maier, C.; Krumova, E.; Scherens, A.; Magerl, W.; Aksu, F.; Zernikow, B. Reference values for quantitative sensory testing in children and adolescents: Developmental and gender differences of somatosensory perception. *Pain* **2010**, *149*, 76–88. [CrossRef] [PubMed]
64. Castien, R.F.; van der Wouden, J.C.; De Hertogh, W. Pressure pain thresholds over the cranio-cervical region in headache: A systematic review and meta-analysis. *J. Headache Pain* **2018**, *19*, 9. [CrossRef] [PubMed]
65. Sollmann, N.; Mathonia, N.; Weidlich, D.; Bonfert, M.; Schroeder, S.A.; Badura, K.A.; Renner, T.; Trepte-Freisleder, F.; Ganter, C.; Krieg, S.M.; et al. Quantitative magnetic resonance imaging of the upper trapezius muscles—Assessment of myofascial trigger points in patients with migraine. *J. Headache Pain* **2019**, *20*, 8. [CrossRef]
66. Sollmann, N.; Schandelmaier, P.; Weidlich, D.; Börner, C.; Urban, G.; Lang, M.; Zimmer, C.; Karampinos, D.C.; Landgraf, M.N.; Heinen, F.; et al. Patients with episodic migraine show increased T2 values of the trapezius muscles—An investigation by quantitative high-resolution magnetic resonance imaging. *Cephalalgia* **2021**, *41*, 934–942. [CrossRef] [PubMed]
67. Edvinsson, L.; Haanes, K.A.; Warfvinge, K. Does inflammation have a role in migraine? *Nat. Rev. Neurol.* **2019**, *15*, 483–490. [CrossRef] [PubMed]

68. Edvinsson, L. Role of CGRP in Migraine. *Handb. Exp. Pharmacol.* **2019**, *255*, 121–130. [CrossRef]
69. Börner, C.; Urban, G.; Beaulieu, L.-D.; Sollmann, N.; Krieg, S.M.; Straube, A.; Renner, T.; Schandelmaier, P.; Lang, M.; Lechner, M., et al. The bottom-up approach: Non-invasive peripheral neurostimulation methods to treat migraine: A scoping review from the child neurologist's perspective. *Eur. J. Paediatr. Neurol.* **2021**, *32*, 16–28. [CrossRef]
70. Lipton, R.B.; Dodick, D.W.; Silberstein, S.D.; Saper, J.R.; Aurora, S.K.; Pearlman, S.H.; E Fischell, R.; Ruppel, P.L.; Goadsby, P.J. Single-pulse transcranial magnetic stimulation for acute treatment of migraine with aura: A randomised, double-blind, parallel-group, sham-controlled trial. *Lancet Neurol.* **2010**, *9*, 373–380. [CrossRef]
71. Stilling, J.M.; Monchi, O.; Amoozegar, F.; Debert, C.T. Transcranial Magnetic and Direct Current Stimulation (TMS/tDCS) for the Treatment of Headache: A Systematic Review. *Headache J. Head Face Pain* **2019**, *59*, 339–357. [CrossRef]
72. Liu, Y.; Dong, Z.; Wang, R.; Ao, R.; Han, X.; Tang, W.; Yu, S. Migraine Prevention Using Different Frequencies of Transcutaneous Occipital Nerve Stimulation: A Randomized Controlled Trial. *J. Pain* **2017**, *18*, 1006–1015. [CrossRef]
73. Magis, D.; Sava, S.; d'Elia, T.S.; Baschi, R.; Schoenen, J. Safety and patients' satisfaction of transcutaneous Supraorbital NeuroStimulation (tSNS) with the Cefaly device in headache treatment: A survey of 2313 headache sufferers in the general population *J. Headache Pain* **2013**, *14*, 95. [CrossRef] [PubMed]
74. Goadsby, P.; Grosberg, B.; Mauskop, A.; Cady, R.; Simmons, K. Effect of noninvasive vagus nerve stimulation on acute migraine: An open-label pilot study. *Cephalalgia* **2014**, *34*, 986–993. [CrossRef] [PubMed]
75. Grazzi, L.; Egeo, G.; Calhoun, A.H.; McClure, C.K.; Liebler, E.; Barbanti, P. Non-invasive Vagus Nerve Stimulation (nVNS) as mini-prophylaxis for menstrual/menstrually related migraine: An open-label study. *J. Headache Pain* **2016**, *17*, 91. [CrossRef] [PubMed]
76. Sampson, M.R.; Benjamin, D.K.; Cohen-Wolkowiez, M. Evidence-based guidelines for pediatric clinical trials: Focus on StaR Child Health. *Expert Rev. Clin. Pharmacol.* **2012**, *5*, 525–531. [CrossRef] [PubMed]
77. Kaptchuk, T.J.; Goldman, P.; A Stone, D.; Stason, W.B. Do medical devices have enhanced placebo effects? *J. Clin. Epidemiology* **2000**, *53*, 786–792. [CrossRef] [PubMed]
78. Steiner, T.J.; Stovner, L.J.; Vos, T.; Jensen, R.; Katsarava, Z. Migraine is first cause of disability in under 50s: Will health politicians now take notice? *J. Headache Pain* **2018**, *19*, 17. [CrossRef]
79. Miller, S.; Matharu, M.S. Migraine is underdiagnosed and undertreated. *Practitioner* **2014**, *258*, 19–24.

children

MDPI

Article

The Real-World Evaluation of Remote Electrical Neuromodulation in Pediatric Migraines: A Preliminary Study

Amit Blumovich [1,2,*], Trevor Gerson [1], Mark Connelly [1], Tammie Wingert [1] and Gina Jones [1]

1 Headache Clinic, Division of Pediatric Neurology, Children's Mercy Hospital, Kansas City, MO 64108, USA; tgerson@cmh.edu (T.G.); mconnelly1@cmh.edu (M.C.); twingert@cmh.edu (T.W.); gljones2@cmh.edu (G.J.)
2 Sackler Faculty of Medicine, Tel Aviv University, Tel Aviv 6997801, Israel
* Correspondence: bluamit@yahoo.com

Abstract

Background/Objectives: Pediatric migraine disrupts school performance and daily functioning. Concerns about medication overuse and limited efficacy highlight the need for non-pharmacologic treatments. The Nerivio remote electrical neuromodulation (REN) device, which is FDA-cleared for ages 8 and above, was evaluated in this study to assess real-world perceptions among patients in a pediatric neurology clinic. **Methods:** Patients aged 10–18 years who had used both acute medications and Nerivio completed two structured questionnaires, one reflecting on experiences with acute medication and one reflecting on experiences with acute REN treatment, assessing school and daily functioning, headache control, medication use, satisfaction, and preference. Descriptive statistics summarized the responses. **Results:** Twenty-four patients participated (91.7% female, mostly aged 13–18 years). Primary outcomes: Nerivio stopped headaches in 33.3% of patients and shortened them in 50.0%, with 41.7% reporting reduced medication use. Exploratory functional outcomes: Missed full school days were unchanged (3.8), partial absences decreased slightly (3.1 to 3.0, ~3%), limited-activity days declined from 3.5 to 2.7 (23%), and days with <50% functioning fell from 4.1 to 3.2 (22%). Preference favored Nerivio in 37.5%, medications in 20.8%, and both equally in 41.7%. Most patients (83.3%) wished to continue; 12.5% reported only mild, transient discomfort, and all continued treatment. **Conclusions:** This preliminary real-world study suggests that REN is feasible and beneficial in pediatric headache care. Primary outcomes demonstrated meaningful headache improvement, while exploratory measures suggested functional gains. REN reduced acute medication use and achieved high satisfaction, supporting its potential role as a patient-centered adjunct in pediatric headache management. Larger studies are needed to confirm these findings.

Keywords: pediatric headache; migraine; remote electrical neuromodulation; Nerivio; acute treatment; non-pharmacologic therapy; real-world evidence

1. Introduction

Migraine and recurrent headache disorders are common in children and adolescents and may substantially interfere with their daily functioning, school performance, and quality of life [1]. Global migraine prevalence estimates reach approximately 8%, underscoring the importance of recognizing the disorder during formative developmental years [2]. In pediatric populations, acute treatment has traditionally relied on over-the-counter (OTC) medications, such as ibuprofen and acetaminophen, which have shown moderate efficacy in randomized trials of children aged $\geq$ 4 years, and their use is supported by international guidelines [3,4]. However, the frequent use of acute migraine medications can contribute to the development of medication overuse headache (MOH) [5], and treatment outcomes are variable. No single therapy for migraine has been shown to be clearly superior, and many patients require tailored interventions when pharmacologic therapy alone is insufficient [6].

Non-pharmacologic approaches, including neuromodulation, are increasingly recognized as promising adjuncts or alternatives for pediatric migraine. The Nerivio device is a remote electrical neuromodulation (REN) wearable that delivers 45 min of controlled electrical stimulation to Aδ and C nerve fibers in the upper arm when a migraine begins, activating conditioned pain modulation pathways that inhibit nociceptive signaling [7,8]. It was initially cleared by the FDA for acute migraine in individuals aged 12 years and older, with more recent clearance extending to children aged 8 years and above. Although pediatric evidence remains limited, prior studies have found that up to 60% of users experience pain relief within two hours, with improvements in functional outcomes and minimal adverse effects [7,8].

While these early studies support the safety and efficacy of REN, less is known about its real-world role alongside standard acute medications in pediatric practice, where treatment decisions are strongly influenced by patient and family experiences. Understanding these real-world, patient-centered perspectives is critical for guiding the adoption and integration of REN into routine migraine management. To address this gap, we undertook a preliminary real-world study aimed at characterizing the clinical and experiential outcomes of Nerivio.

2. Materials and Methods

This project was conducted at the Pediatric Neurology Clinic of Children's Mercy Hospital, a tertiary care center in Kansas City, MO, USA, from 3 March to 30 June 2025. Eligible participants were children and adolescents aged 10–18 years with a clinical diagnosis of migraine, according to the International Classification of Headache Disorders (ICHD-3) criteria, who were using both over-the-counter (OTC) acute medications and the Nerivio device (Theranica Bio-Electronics Ltd., Netanya, Israel) for migraine treatment. Patients were recruited during routine neurology follow-up visits. All participants had previously used over-the-counter (OTC) acute medications before initiating Nerivio and were maintained on stable preventive regimens throughout the study period. The questionnaires were completed at a single timepoint, based on participants' retrospective reports after they had gained experience with both treatments, ensuring consistent recall.

Data were collected using two structured questionnaires. The "acute medications" questionnaire assessed headache characteristics, school absences, functional disability, medication response, and satisfaction with acute pharmacologic therapy. The "acute treatment with REN" questionnaire evaluated perceived changes in headache burden, school attendance, activity limitation, medication use, and treatment satisfaction. In the REN questionnaire, patients were also asked to describe their perceived treatment effects using predefined categories: "stopped headache" (complete resolution of pain within two hours after stimulation), "shortened headache" ($\geq$50% reduction in attack duration compared with typical episodes), and "less medication" (a subjective patient-reported decrease in the frequency or amount of acute medication used after starting Nerivio).

Information on the number of acute Nerivio treatments per participant was not systematically recorded; therefore, findings primarily reflect general real-world impressions following limited exposure to REN.

Questionnaires were initially distributed electronically through a REDCap-based clinical registry (Research Electronic Data Capture; Vanderbilt University, Nashville, TN, USA); however, due to low response rates, subsequent data were collected on paper during clinic visits. Participation was voluntary, and responses were anonymized.

Functional outcomes, including missed school days, reduced activity, and impaired functioning, were adapted from the Pediatric Migraine Disability Assessment (PedMIDAS), a validated instrument for measuring headache-related disability in pediatric populations. Because both questionnaires were completed concurrently for patients with prior documented use of both treatments, PedMIDAS items were used descriptively rather than as longitudinal measures. To align with the retrospective design, participants were asked to report functioning over a recent representative period rather than the original three-month PedMIDAS timeframe.

Descriptive statistics were used to summarize categorical responses and to estimate mean values for ordinal ranges (e.g., 1–2 days, 3–5 days). Results are presented as absolute values, mean changes, and percent reductions, which serve as effect size estimates to illustrate the magnitude and direction of change. Comparisons between baseline and post-Nerivio periods were descriptive; no formal inferential statistics were applied given the exploratory design and limited sample size. Data were visualized using bar charts and comparative plots.

3. Results

3.1. Study Population

A total of 24 pediatric patients diagnosed with migraine according to the International Classification of Headache Disorders (ICHD-3), aged 10–18 years, were included. Most (87.5%) were in the 13–18-year-old age group, and 91.7% identified as female. This distribution reflects the well-documented higher prevalence of migraine in female adolescents and the randomized nature of the questionnaire distribution within the clinic. All participants reported a long-standing history of migraine attacks, typically lasting either 1–6 h or more than 24 h (Figure 1).

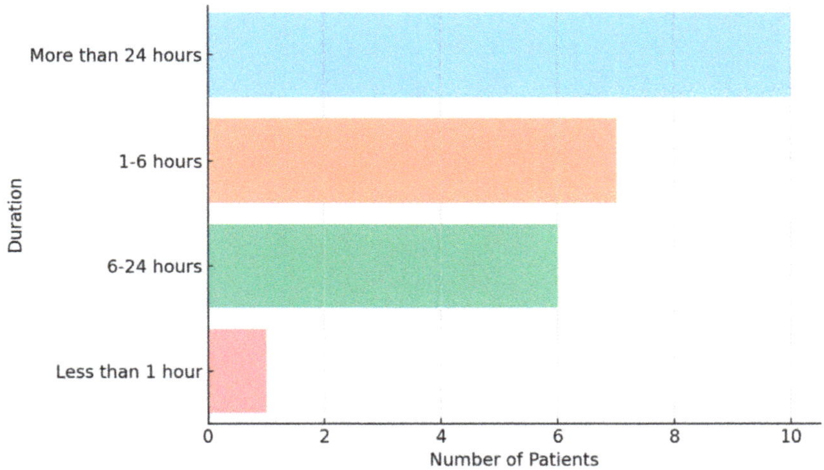

Figure 1. Distribution of headache episode duration reported prior to Nerivio use.

3.2. Treatment Effectiveness and Medication Reduction

When asked about the specific effects of Nerivio, 8 out of 24 patients (33.3%) reported that it "stopped the headache". A further 12 out of 24 respondents (50.0%) indicated that it "shortened the headache," and 10 out of 24 participants (41.7%) reported a reduced need for acute medications after Nerivio use (Figure 2).

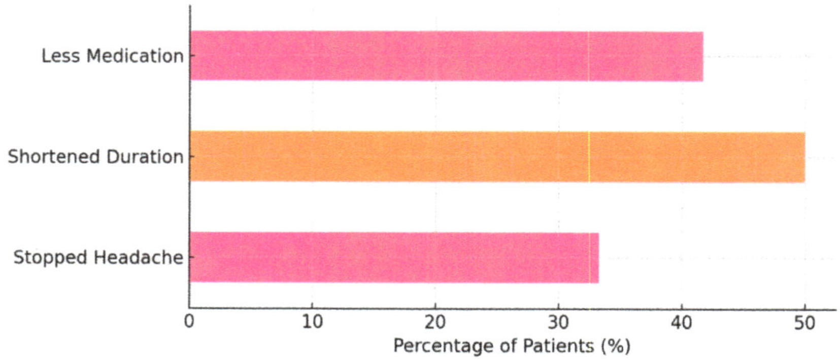

Figure 2. Percentage of patients reporting clinical benefit from Nerivio use.

3.3. Functional Outcomes Before and After Nerivio Use

Functional limitations due to headache were evaluated based on responses to the acute medication and REN questionnaires, reflecting retrospective reports of patients who had used both treatments. This design captured real-world perceptions of acute effects rather than preventive outcomes. Accordingly, functional data were summarized descriptively rather than interpreted as preventive effects. The average number of missed full school days remained stable at 3.8 days. Missed partial school days decreased slightly from 3.1 to 3.0 days (~3% reduction). Days for which other activities (e.g., play, sports) were stopped declined from 3.5 to 2.7 (23% reduction), and days with functioning at <50% ability decreased from 4.1 to 3.2 (22% reduction). Formal statistical testing was not performed given the sample size and preliminary design (Figure 3).

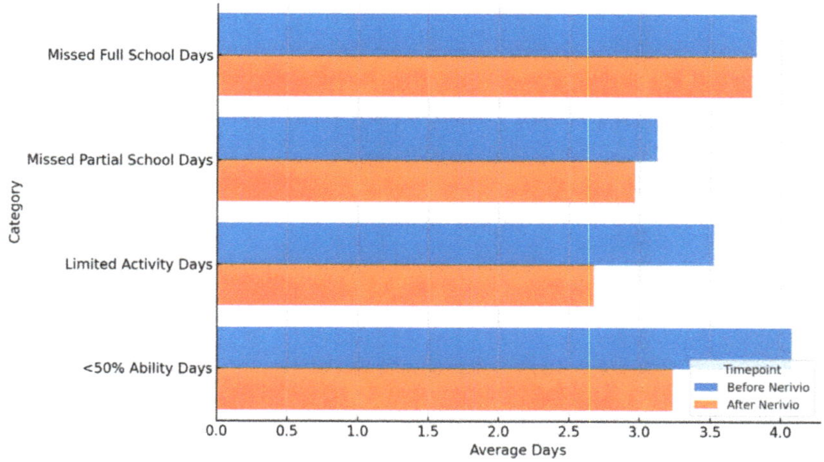

Figure 3. Mean number of days with missed school, reduced activity, and impaired function before vs. after Nerivio treatment.

3.4. Treatment Preference

Treatment preference responses favored Nerivio in 9 of 24 patients (37.5%) and favored medications in 5 of 24 cases (20.8%). Patients demonstrated an equal preference for both treatments in 10 out of 24 cases (41.7%) (Figure 4).

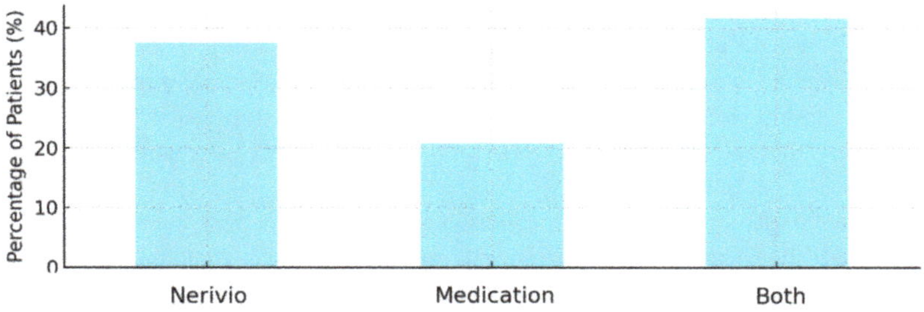

Figure 4. Patient preference for Nerivio vs. medications.

3.5. Satisfaction and Tolerability

Most patients (20/24, 83.3%) expressed a willingness to continue using Nerivio. Three patients (12.5%) reported mild discomfort (e.g., local tingling or tightness at the stimulation site). All participants continued treatment despite these discomforts, which were consistent with expected device-related sensations (Figure 5).

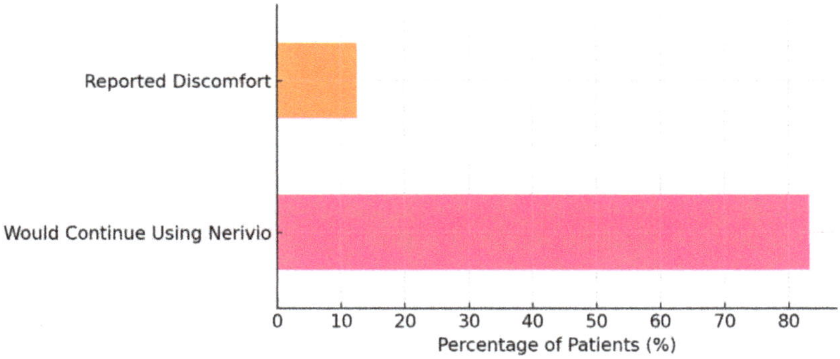

Figure 5. Percentage of patients reporting satisfaction and discomfort with Nerivio.

4. Discussion

This preliminary study evaluated real-world patient experiences with Nerivio, a wearable remote electrical neuromodulation (REN) device, in the context of routine pediatric headache management. Consistent with prior clinical and real-world studies of REN [7,8], our findings provide preliminary evidence on functional outcomes, treatment satisfaction, and patient preferences in children and adolescents with migraine.

Although the average number of missed full school days in our cohort remained unchanged, Nerivio use was associated with fewer partial absences and a reduction in days with limited activity and <50% functioning. These exploratory functional findings parallel prior REN studies demonstrating decreased functional disability during migraine attacks [7,8] and align with broader evidence that non-pharmacologic interventions—including cognitive behavioral therapy, which has been shown to reduce headache days and migraine-related disability in children [9], and psychologically based approaches such as relaxation and biofeedback [10]—can support daily functioning and school attendance in pediatric populations with migraine.

As the primary outcomes, a large proportion of patients reported meaningful headache benefits with REN, including complete cessation in one-third and shortened durations in about one-half of participants. These findings also align with clinical trial data showing 58.9–74.2% pain relief and 20.0–35.6% pain freedom at 2 h [7], as well as adolescent trial findings of 71% pain relief and 35% pain freedom [8]. Importantly, 41.7% of patients required less acute medication after using Nerivio, supporting the potential of REN as a medication-sparing strategy [7,8]. This is particularly relevant in pediatric populations, where medication overuse headache, tolerability issues, and caregiver concerns remain persistent challenges [5,6].

Treatment preference results in our cohort varied, with a little over one-third favoring Nerivio, one-fifth favoring medication, and the remainder reporting equal benefits. This heterogeneity underscores the individualized nature of migraine care and reinforces the importance of offering a range of therapeutic options tailored to patient and family priorities. Nerivio tolerability was favorable, with only 12.5% of patients reporting discomfort and the majority (83.3%) expressing a willingness to continue use. Reported discomfort was mild and transient, described mainly as brief tingling or tightness at the application site, and all participants continued the treatment despite these sensations. These findings are consistent with prior REN safety data [7,8] and support the device's integration as a non-pharmacologic adjunct in clinical practice.

Several limitations should be noted. The small sample size, single-site design, and reliance on self-reported outcomes limit generalizability and introduce a potential reporting bias. Because both acute medications and acute treatment with REN questionnaires were completed during the same visit, this study reflects retrospective perceptions rather than longitudinal outcomes, and therefore preventive or causal effects cannot be inferred. Detailed frequency data on headache episodes and acute medication use before and after Nerivio initiation were not systematically collected, as the study emphasized patients' perceived experiences and real-world impressions of treatment efficacy. Additionally, some participants may have continued using acute medications alongside REN, which could partially confound treatment attributions. Finally, analyses were descriptive and exploratory, aimed at illustrating effect size trends rather than testing statistical significance.

Despite these limitations, this study contributes to the body of growing evidence that demonstrates that REN is feasible, acceptable, and potentially beneficial in pediatric migraine care. It highlights the importance of incorporating patient-reported experiences into evaluations of new therapies and suggests that REN may reduce functional disability and reliance on acute medications in everyday practice. Future research with larger, more diverse samples and controlled designs will be critical to confirm these findings and to guide the integration of REN into pediatric headache management pathways.

5. Conclusions

In this preliminary real-world study, the Nerivio REN device demonstrated meaningful clinical benefits for pediatric patients with migraine, with primary outcomes showing headache improvement and exploratory measures suggesting potential functional gains. Most patients expressed satisfaction, and more than 80% reported a willingness to continue use, underscoring the device's acceptability in routine care. Although these findings are based on retrospective patient reports from a small, single-site sample, they support the feasibility and potential clinical value of REN as a patient-centered, non-pharmacologic adjunct in pediatric headache management.

Author Contributions: Conceptualization, A.B., T.G., M.C. and G.J.; methodology, A.B., T.G., M.C. and G.J.; investigation, A.B., T.G. and T.W.; data curation, A.B.; formal analysis, A.B.; writing—original draft preparation, A.B.; writing—review and editing, T.G., M.C., T.W. and G.J.; supervision, G.J. All authors have read and agreed to the published version of the manuscript.

Funding: This research received no external funding.

Institutional Review Board Statement: This project was reviewed by the hospital's Office of Research Integrity and was determined not to meet the definition of human participant research under 45 CFR 46.102(l). Therefore, Institutional Review Board approval was not required.

Informed Consent Statement: Not applicable. This project was determined not to meet the definition of human participant research; therefore, informed consent was not required under institutional policies.

Data Availability Statement: De-identified questionnaire data and the aggregated dataset used for analysis are available from the corresponding author upon reasonable request. Individual patient-level data cannot be shared publicly to protect privacy.

Acknowledgments: During the manuscript preparation, the authors used generative artificial intelligence (GenAI) for assistance with the preparation of graphs. All outputs were reviewed and verified by the authors, who take full responsibility for the accuracy and integrity of the manuscript.

Conflicts of Interest: Dr. Gerson received an honorarium from Theranica for participation in a past advisory board. The other authors declare no conflicts of interest.

References

1. Powers, S.W.; Patton, S.R.; Hommel, K.A.; Hershey, A.D. Quality of life in childhood migraines: Clinical impact and comparison to other chronic illnesses. *Pediatrics* **2003**, *112*, e1–e5. [CrossRef] [PubMed]
2. Abu-Arafeh, I.; Razak, S.; Sivaraman, B.; Graham, C. Prevalence of headache and migraine in children and adolescents: A systematic review of population-based studies. *Dev. Med. Child Neurol.* **2010**, *52*, 1088–1097. [CrossRef] [PubMed]
3. Hämäläinen, M.L.; Hoppu, K.; Valkeila, E.; Santavuori, P. Ibuprofen or acetaminophen for the acute treatment of migraine in children: A double blind, randomized, placebo controlled, crossover study. *Neurology* **1997**, *48*, 103–107. [CrossRef] [PubMed]
4. Oskoui, M.; Pringsheim, T.; Holler-Managan, Y.; Potrebic, S.; Billinghurst, L.; Gloss, D.; Hershey, A.D.; Licking, N.; Sowell, M.; Victorio, M.C.; et al. Practice guideline update summary: Acute treatment of migraine in children and adolescents. *Neurology* **2019**, *93*, 487–499. [CrossRef] [PubMed]
5. Diener, H.C.; Holle, D.; Solbach, K.; Gaul, C. Medication overuse headache: Risk factors, pathophysiology and management. *Nat. Rev. Neurol.* **2016**, *12*, 575–583. [CrossRef] [PubMed]
6. VanderPluym, J.H.; Cheng, N.; Zhu, Y.; Wang, Z.; Morris, C.; Jones, A.; Gelfand, A.A.; Gautreaux, J. Treatment of medication overuse headache in children and adolescents: A systematic review. *Headache* **2025**, *65*, 1148–1159. [CrossRef] [PubMed]
7. Tepper, S.J.; Lin, T.; Montal, T.; Ironi, A.; Dougherty, C. Real world experience with remote electrical neuromodulation in the acute treatment of migraine. *Pain Med.* **2020**, *21*, 3522–3529. [CrossRef] [PubMed]
8. Hershey, A.D.; Lin, T.; Gruper, Y.; Harris, D.; Ironi, A.; Berk, T.; Szperka, C.L.; Berenson, F. Remote electrical neuromodulation for acute treatment of migraine in adolescents. *Headache* **2021**, *61*, 310–317. [CrossRef] [PubMed]
9. Powers, S.W.; Kashikar-Zuck, S.M.; Allen, J.R.; LeCates, S.L.; Slater, S.K.; Zafar, M.; Kabbouche, M.A.; O'Brien, H.L.; Shenk, C.E.; Rausch, J.R.; et al. Cognitive behavioral therapy plus amitriptyline for chronic migraine in children and adolescents: A randomized clinical trial. *JAMA* **2013**, *310*, 2622–2630. [CrossRef] [PubMed]
10. Trautmann, E.; Lackschewitz, H.; Kröner-Herwig, B. Psychological treatment of recurrent headache in children and adolescents: A meta-analysis. *Cephalalgia* **2006**, *26*, 1411–1426. [CrossRef] [PubMed]

children

MDPI

Review

Chronic Pediatric Headache as a Manifestation of Shunt Over-Drainage and Slit Ventricle Syndrome in Patients Harboring a Cerebrospinal Fluid Diversion System: A Narrative Literature Review

Dimitrios Panagopoulos [1,*], Maro Gavra [2], Efstathios Boviatsis [3], Stefanos Korfias [4] and Marios Themistocleous [1]

1 Neurosurgical Department, Pediatric Hospital of Athens, 45701 Athens, Greece; mthemistocleous@gmail.com
2 Neuro-Radiology Department, Pediatric Hospital of Athens, 45701 Athens, Greece; mmgavra@yahoo.com
3 2nd University Neurosurgical Department, Medical School, General Hospital of Athens 'Attikon', University of Athens, 12462 Athens, Greece; eboviatsis@gmail.com
4 1st University Neurosurgical Department, Medical School, General Hospital of Athens 'Evangelismos', University of Athens, 10676 Athens, Greece; skorfias@otenet.gr
* Correspondence: dimpanayop@gmail.com

Abstract: The main subject of the current review is a specific subtype of headache, which is related to shunt over-drainage and slit ventricle syndrome, in pediatric patients harboring an implanted shunt device for the management of hydrocephalus. This clinical entity, along with its impairment regarding the quality of life of the affected individuals, is generally underestimated. This is partly due to the absence of universally agreed-upon diagnostic criteria, as well as due to a misunderstanding of the interactions among the implicated pathophysiological mechanisms. A lot of attempts have been performed to propose an integrative model, aiming at the determination of all the offending mechanisms of the shunt over-drainage syndrome, as well as the determination of all the clinical characteristics and related symptomatology that accompany these secondary headaches. This subcategory of headache, named postural dependent headache, can be associated with nausea, vomiting, and/or radiological signs of slim ventricles and/or subdural collections. The ultimate goal of our review is to draw clinicians' attention, especially that of those that are managing pediatric patients with permanent, long-standing, ventriculoperitoneal, or, less commonly, ventriculoatrial shunts. We attempted to elucidate all clinical and neurological characteristics that are inherently related to this type of headache, as well as to highlight the current management options. This specific subgroup of patients may eventually suffer from severe, intractable headaches, which may negatively impair their quality of daily living. In the absence of any other clinical condition that could be incriminated as the cause of the headache, shunt over-drainage should not be overlooked. On the contrary, it should be seriously taken into consideration, and its management should be added to the therapeutic armamentarium of such cases, which are difficult to be handled.

Keywords: over-drainage; slit ventricle syndrome; anti-siphon device; programmable valve

1. Introduction

A recently published meta-analysis, centered on the epidemiological features of pediatric primary headache, estimated that the approximate incidence of migraine in the pediatric and adolescent population overall is in the area of 11% [1]. According to published series, the incidence of pediatric headache varies among the different subgroup of patients, based on their age. Namely, it is more pronounced in children aged approximately 13 years of age [2]. It is worthwhile to mention that headaches are subdivided as primary—that is, of unknown etiology—and secondary, which are intimately related to a relevant pathophysiologic substrate [1]. Among these subtypes of headaches, the headache that accompanies shunt over-drainage and slit ventricle syndrome deserves special mention. The exact frequency of shunt over-drainage postural headache in the pediatric population is unknown as it is difficult to quantify an entity that entails only quality characteristics.

Another parameter that needs to be underlined is that the treatment options are restricted as the pathophysiology that accompanies this spectrum of disorders is not fully elucidated. The main reason for this confusion comes from the limited number of relevant, detailed epidemiological surveys dedicated to the prevalence and incidence of primary headaches in the pediatric age group [1,2]. Moreover, the existing ones are frequently heterogeneous, and this is an intimate characteristic of the intrinsic characteristics of the studies [2,3]. These include age range, sex, social and economic background, the utilized methodologies (e.g., school-based questionnaires, clinician interviews, phone surveys), along with the different inclusion criteria applied, which occasionally could not be considered specific to developmental age [3]. So, when a comparison is attempted with headaches in their adult counterparts, especially due to all of these restrictions, a limited number of epidemiological studies are available in children and adolescents. Namely, based on bibliographic data, the estimated prevalence of headache and migraine is up to 58% and 7.7% [4], respectively. In children and adolescents, their quality of life is substantially impaired by headaches, causing negative feedback in their daily living [5], i.e., the elimination of their social activities and physical activity, school absenteeism, weaker learning outcomes, a higher risk of dropping out of school, and a negative effect on parent's careers [5,6].

The main purpose of this review is to analyze a subcategory of pediatric headaches that arise as a secondary effect to the iatrogenic management of pediatric hydrocephalus. We have collected relevant data regarding chronic shunt over-drainage and slit ventricle syndrome and have tried to investigate their pathophysiological association with the development of secondary headaches, which are often refractory to medical treatment.

2. Materials and Methods

Search Strategy

We executed a title-specific search using PubMed as well as the Thomson Reuters Web of Science database to identify the articles (reviews, case reports, original research, technical notes) that were related to shunt over-drainage, slit ventricle syndrome, and headache with respect to ependymomas and other posterior fossa tumors (as these patients frequently harbor a ventriculoperitoneal shunt). The time range of our search was extended from 1968—when, to the best of our knowledge, the first bibliographic report on shunt over-drainage appeared—to March 2024. A specific age range was included as a selection criterion; more precisely, our search included only data that were extracted from patients under 18 years of age. Afterwards, we reviewed the results in order to clarify that they were relevant for the purposes of our research. The papers that were chosen were further analyzed in order to extract any conclusions regarding the existence of any association between shunt over-drainage and slit ventricle syndrome and a headache that is resistant to all conservative treatment modalities.

3. Discussion

3.1. Shunt Over-Drainage and Its Association with Headache

The term shunt over-drainage is utilized in order to delimit a well-known complication that is causally related to excessive drainage of cerebrospinal fluid in patients harboring a CSF shunt system. The term "over-drainage" was first utilized in bibliographic series in 1968 [7,8] and has been increasingly accepted and adopted since the 1990s [9,10]. It is widely known that over-drainage represents one of the most frequently encountered complications that is secondary to CSF shunting procedures [11]. It may be associated with all types of CSF diversion procedures and is not restricted to any specific pediatric age-group but is most-commonly encountered with valve-bearing shunt systems [12]. The clinical equivalent of this pathology is named postural headache and is manifested radiologically with a slender ventricular system ("slit ventricle syndrome"). Due to the common coexistence of these two entities, postural headache is currently being considered as a clinical observation that is frequently recorded in combination with over-drainage [13–16]. Shunt over-drainage could be combined with different clinical and radiological features, such as subdural hygroma [13,17–19] and premature closure of cranial sutures (in infants) [9,20], as well as low ICP syndrome [21]. All of these manifestations should be integrated under the umbrella of shunt over-drainage. There is a wide discrepancy regarding the estimated prevalence of the precise incidence of over-drainage according to current literature data, as it varies from 2 to 71%. The most accepted explanation for this marked fluctuation regarding the statements for this syndrome could be based upon the non-well-specified diagnostic criteria, the heterogeneity of the investigated populations, and the different policies for follow-up after shunting [15,16,22]. Moreover, it is also corroborated that over-drainage may be under-reported, and thus underestimated, due to the lack of consensus regarding the definition criteria of this entity, as well as due to an incomplete knowledge of pathophysiology [16,23]. Consistent with our statements is a survey that was executed among American pediatric neurosurgeons, which documents the lack of consent and the existing uncertainty regarding the understanding and management of over-drainage-associated complications [22]. Apart from that, the range of normal reference values regarding ICP and probably postural CSF pressure/volume regulation seem to be intimately related to age. All of these data imply that the risk of over-drainage, its clinical manifestations, treatment modalities, and protocols may not follow the same pattern in pediatric and adult cohorts. Moreover, this may also be true when toddlers and young teenagers are under investigation [24–27]. The majority of researchers agree that the remarkable variability regarding the estimated incidence that is referred to in published data is intimately related to the lack of a widely accepted definition [24–27]. This ultimately results in the absence a of clinical consensus and doubtfulness about diagnosis.

3.2. Evolution of Concepts and Current Pitfalls in Shunt Over-Drainage Syndrome

There are several premature—even sparse—previously reported bibliographic reports of inappropriate over-drainage of cerebrospinal fluid in the form of anecdotal cases [8,16,28–33]. Fox and coworkers [34] were the first who attempted to record ICP monitoring data in shunted patients. Their data were extracted from 18 patients suffering from normal pressure hydrocephalus; their relevant mean cerebrospinal fluid pressure values were about −220 mm H_2O for ventriculoperitoneal shunts and about −190 mm H_2O for ventriculoarterial shunts when they were assuming an upright position. These findings were initially attributed to the siphoning effect of shunts. The initial management option that was adopted was the incorporation of higher-pressure valves, along with VAS, especially for patients who are expected to adopt an upright posture for the majority of their waking period [8]. Portnoy contributed to this "mechanistic model" by developing an antisiphon device, aiming at the prevention of the effect of siphoning [31,35]. ICP characteristics of siphoning related to postural changes were confirmed in 1990 by Chapman, who utilized a telemetric device in patients with VPS, VAS, and ventriculopleural shunts. Initial investigations centered on the definition of the role of ASD revealed that they were, in general terms, effective in the restoration of "normal pressures" in the upright position [36].

3.3. Clinical Manifestations in Shunt Over-Drainage Postural Headache

The clinical manifestations of over-drainage of CSF may be present in an acute pattern, and this complication is not intimately related to the development of chronic refractory headaches [37,38]. A minority of patients may not even manifest any symptomatology after the adoption of low values of intracranial pressure [39]. When a constellation of symptoms appears, they more commonly consist of a "low-pressure headache", i.e., a headache that is intimately associated with the patient's posture or "spinal headache". This is clinically manifested with the patient being unable to assume an upright position. The constellation of symptoms may also include nuchal or upper back pain, nausea, vomiting, dizziness, fatigue, irritability, gait disturbance, diplopia, seizures, and lethargy [40,41]. Symptomatology associated with low intracranial pressure may eventually evolve to intermittent disabling headaches. The next step in the evolution of this clinical syndrome is related to chronic pathological entities, which include developmental delay, decline in school performance, and social withdrawal. When the clinical records of these patients are carefully reviewed, multiple episodes of shunt revisions are frequently registered, which are in accordance with episodes of severe and intractable headaches.

3.4. Sequale of Over-Drainage

The conception of excessive drainage of CSF was presented by Dandy in 1932. In 1968, Becker et al. utilized the term "over-drainage" in order to explain the pathophysiologic substrate of the mechanism by which the over-drainage can induce depression of the fontanelle, as well as overriding sutures, craniosynostosis, low ventricular pressure, and, finally, small ventricles [7,8]. This sequence of events involves only the infant population. Pudenz et al. first published a review article centered on over-drainage that was causally related to insertion of a shunt device in 1991 [10]; they concluded that premature closure of cranial sutures and skull deformities (in infants), stenosis or occlusion of the aqueduct, SVS, and low-ICP syndrome are all included in the constellation of manifestations that constitute over-drainage.

In 2018, Ros et al. published a review centered on shunt over-drainage syndrome, attempting to specify the constellation of clinical characteristics that constitute over-drainage. These include headache, with or without associated vomiting and neurological signs or symptoms, plus different degrees of altered consciousness in association with the radiological evidence of small ventricular size and subdural collections of blood or fluid [15]. Current evidence suggests that over-drainage can manifest with a broad spectrum of clinical manifestations; these could include postural headache, subdural hygromas/hematomas, stenosis/occlusion of the aqueduct of Sylvius, craniosynostosis, SVS (characterized by intermittent headache, small ventricles, and slow refilling of the ventricular shunt reservoir), and obstruction of the ventricular catheter. Even though the concept of "over-drainage" has been identified as an adverse effect related to the surgical management of hydrocephalus for several decades, the absence of a strict circumscription, as well as consistent terminology to delineate the concept of over-drainage based on bibliographic reports, is conspicuous.

3.5. Prevention of Headaches Associated with Shunt Over-Drainage: A Brief Summary of Existing Data Regarding Their Pathophysiology, Clinical Symptoms, Treatment, and Prevention

According to a recently published data base [42,43], in about 3% of cases that necessitated a shunt revision procedure, the underlying pathophysiologic mechanism was recorded to be excessive CSF drainage. Nevertheless, the actual relevant rate is rather underestimated, with experts raising this percentage to the rate of 20% of cases. Several techniques aiming towards the reduction of the rate of CSF drainage have been described, incorporating the use of high-pressure non-programmable fixed differential pressure valves, flow valves, and programmable differential pressure valves [11,44,45]. A major drawback that is inherently associated with these cases is related to the fact that CSF drainage may not be as is required when the patient assumes a vertical posture. On the contrary, any attempt to solely increase the differential pressure of the valves was not associated with encouraging results in several published series [11,44,46,47]. These observations forced scientists to develop new mechanistic models related to the pattern of shunt drainage protocols. The main representative of these newly developed drainage systems was included under the umbrella of antisiphon systems. The main aim associated with their development was the prevention of gravitational-related over pull of CSF when the patient is attempting the upright posture. The common concept that underlies the function of antisiphon systems is that they are supposed to be able to adapt to alternating clinical situations or physical conditions, such as the change from the supine to the erect posture [11,48].

Another pathophysiologic mechanism that is inherently related to the development of intractable headaches, especially in the pediatric population, is related to the concept of the slit ventricle syndrome. This is widely recognized as one of the potential side effects of CSF over-drainage, and its pathophysiologic explanation is primarily associated with the acquisition of a pathologically diminished cerebral compliance with a typical leftward shift of the curve in the pressure/volume graph. The collapsed ventricular configuration represents the most typical radiographic feature of SVS. This feature by no means could be considered as been pathognomonic of SVS, as many patients may not exhibit any clinical symptoms. The exact prevalence of a collapsed ventricular system is not universally accepted, although it has been reported in the range of 10–85% of all shunted patients [49]. A wide variety of clinical symptoms have been related to SVS, and a world-wide unanimity regarding its definition does not exist. Nevertheless, classic SVS clinical features consist of severe and persistent or recurrent headaches, frequently related to or provoked by positional changes. The constellation of symptoms, apart from headaches, include vomiting, weakness, ataxia, seizures, cranial nerve deficit, bradycardia, and systemic hypertension, especially in more compromised patients [50,51]. The referring physicians have attempted several positional changes, along with valve upgrade as recommended by several literature reviews [52–55]. Several patients have undergone repeated procedures aiming toward valve replacement (using valves without any antisiphon system). Nevertheless, none of these interventions have provided permanent relief of the symptomatology of the affected individual.

Apart from small ventricular size, patients suffering from SVS may present with several indirect radiologic signs of over-drainage. These include a small-sized posterior fossa, hyperostosis of the calvarium, dolichocephalic disproportion, suture sclerosis in proximity to the skull base, parenchymal calcifications, and/or sinus hyperpneumatization [56–58]. MRI may prove to be a useful diagnostic modality, as it may offer valuable details about the ventricular and cistern anatomy [52,59–61]. Relevant—albeit not usual—MRI findings include the existence of epidural venous plexus engorgement [52,62], along with lumbar canal stenosis [11,63,64]. Other anecdotally reported findings include the existence of pneumocephalus, as well as isolated ventricles [64], along with extra-axial collections of fluid or blood [51,65–67].

The proposed treatment algorithm for these groups of patients varies greatly [68,69]. Regarding the less-severe cases, the current trend is the selection of a conservative management protocol [52–55]. In general terms, the management of SVS should aim to restore the pathologically reduced cerebral compliance. Several treatment modalities have been proposed, thus reflecting the inhomogeneity and complexity of the implicated pathophysiologic mechanisms, as no one individual pathogenetic theory could explain the wide variety of clinical manifestations of this syndrome. Other treatment modalities, such as ETV, lumbar drainage, and cranial expansion, have been utilized in refractory cases [70]. Nevertheless, the treatment of SVS may be associated with a wide range of complications and failures to manage it successfully; the exact prevalence of all these complications is unclear as the relevant literature is mainly based on case reports rather than clinical series [51,70,71].

3.6. Management of SVS: A Brief Summary of Management Protocols, Including Our Clinical Experience

The most commonly utilized therapeutic measurement, as the first step of our treatment algorithm regarding SVS, is related to upgrading the valve to higher opening pressure values. Although it is technically easy, the overall handling of cases that are managed in such a manner is generally demanding [71,72]. The clinical experience that we have gained with the management of such cases has pointed out the significance of the incremental titration of the valve pressure settings, which means that one level setting adjustment at a time is the only safe and acceptable strategy. According to most centers' recorded data, this option offers the most effective alleviation of the relevant symptomatology in the greater percentage of individuals who are suffering from a mild range of symptoms. This is especially true for the pediatric cohort of patients, and this seems to be due to the lesser disturbance of the curvature that follows the cerebral compliance as the time course of the disease is sooner and the diagnosis is relatively earlier registered. On the contrary, we have realized that the more severe or more chronic the clinical equivalent of the syndrome, the lesser the chances that a positive and long-lasting response will occur or, more importantly, will be permanent. Reinforcing this view is the fact that it is based on a recent relevant study [42], which enrolled a subgroup of 16 patients that were severely affected and who were improved by valve reprogramming.

Another subgroup of patients has failed these conservative measurements, and it requires surgical treatment. The current trend is to initially attempt externalization of the existent shunt. This therapeutic manipulation offers us the opportunity to obtain valuable and measurable evidence of the initial opening pressure, as well as the possibility to monitor the fluctuations of the ICP values. These variations in the measurements of ICP could be used as guidance when we attempt to increase the reservoir height. There are reports that have proposed that the spontaneous ICP fluctuations, along with the ICP variations to consecutive alterations of reservoir height, could be considered as the mainstay for the invention of the ongoing management options [38]. Several relevant studies [73–76] have adopted a treatment protocol, which is based upon the ICP values. More precisely, when individuals manifesting with normal or high ICP are being managed, even when the ventricular system is considered to be small, the initial management option was direct shunt replacement using programmable differential pressure valves, which incorporated an antisiphon system. On the other hand, for patients with low ICP measurements, an EVD was the treatment modality of choice. Following that, the ICP gradually increased by a progressive increasement of the reservoir height. For these patients who demonstrated ventricular enlargement concurrently with an increase in ICP values, the proposed management option was an ETV, based on the hypothesis that it could restore the cerebral compliance towards normal values and equilibrate the pressure gradient between ventricles and subarachnoid spaces. There are reports that support the efficacy of this treatment modality [76].

Another subgroup of patients includes those cases which demonstrate a ventricular system whose dimensions remained unchanged, despite the increases in ICP measurements. They received a new programmable differential pressure valve, with an incorporated antisiphon system. There are data which support that upgrading of the valve opening pressure obviated the need for—or at least delayed—surgical intervention in one third of cases. Moreover, according to published studies, an initial attempt based on conservative treatment constitutes a reasonable suggestion [44,69,75,77]. It is widely accepted that young patients' age and the utilization of an antisiphon system are factors that are associated with a significantly favorable outcome.

In conclusion, we have mentioned several studies which state that VPS replacement constitutes the optimum therapeutic option for SVS; the simultaneous incorporation of an antisiphon device and valve substitution is strongly recommended [11,44,47,48].

In the subgroup of patients who share a significantly reduced cerebral compliance, it could be beneficial to incorporate a programmable antisiphon system in conjunction with the valvular mechanism. This combination offers the capability of gradually modifying either the ICP or the drainage modalities, or even both of them [11,44,48].

3.7. Clinical and Radiologic Outcome

Even though there is a considerable addition of knowledge regarding SVS, as well as technical improvements in the embiomechanics of the shunt systems, the overall natural history of SVS continues to be unpredictable in a vast majority of patients. According to a recently published series [42], no more than half of the participants demonstrated complete resolution of their findings in terms of clinical and radiologic improvement. We would like to mention once more that children were associated with significantly better outcomes than their adult counterparts, and a negative association is established as patient's age increases.

A major drawback when our therapeutic armamentarium regarding SVS treatment has been considered is related to the fact that most cases have been anecdotally reported, and large case series with previously reporting specific results and treatment outcomes are lacking [15,42]. Current treatment targets are mainly centered on the control of CSF over-drainage and on the improvement of cerebral compliance.

We have concluded that patients suffering from hydrocephalus who have initially been treated with a programmable differential pressure valve were associated with a lesser chance of developing SVS. Nevertheless, it seems that the initial placement of antisiphon systems could not provide any protective effect against the development of SVS.

There is consensus that prompt, proper, and, eventually, a more aggressive treatment may lead to better control of the syndrome in all age-groups.

Another important notice is related to the fact that an immediate and appropriate diagnosis is of inherently significant importance. This is explained by the assumption that a protracted clinical course stands for more protracted periods with negatively impaired quality of life. The current trend stands for the importance of the utilization of valves that offer more options for non-invasive interventions, as well as shunt systems that are an integral part of more sophisticated programmable valves. These options could offer a new therapeutic armamentarium in our attempt to attain the prevention and management of this entity. Apart from that, SVS constitutes a challenging problem, and we have to assume that all treatments modalities have failed in a significant percentage of patients. We hope that ongoing technical innovations will essentially aid in the prevention, diagnosis, and treatment of SVS.

In conclusion, the pathophysiologic entities of shunt over-drainage and slit ventricle syndrome should always be included in our differential diagnostic plan whenever we are confronted with intractable headaches that may resemble the inherent characteristics of migraine in a patient who harbors a ventriculoperitoneal or a ventriculoatrial shunt, especially from infancy. In cases where the diagnostic work-up is unable to underline another pathological substrate, we should maintain the suspicion that our patient could fulfill the diagnostic criteria necessary to be considered under the umbrella of shunt over-drainage and slit ventricle syndrome.

The following table (Table 1) presents a proposed treatment and diagnostic algorithm in cases of chronic headache in pediatric patients suffering from SVS. We would like to clarify that this is an algorithm proposed by the authors based on literature data and their clinical experience.

From our perspective, the overall benefit with this article to the readers is its highlighting the importance of the recognition by the scientific community of the type of headache that is related to shunt over-drainage and slit ventricle syndrome, which is secondary to the surgical management of pediatric hydrocephalus, especially in infants. Excessive CSF drainage following the insertion of a ventricular shunt is a well-known complication that is intimately related to the treatment of hydrocephalus. Nevertheless, the absence of a widely accepted definition in the literature is evident, as well as its consequences. There is no consensus regarding the relevant diagnostic criteria, and, because of this, the exact incidence remains unknown. The overall impact of this uncertainty is reflected in the absence of recommendations dedicated to the prevention, management, and treatment of this condition. Since no consensus has been achieved for several decades, we strongly consider that a definition of OD should not be based upon individual but separate opinions;instead, a significant degree of agreement should be achieved by the majority of OD specialists.

Table 1. Proposed treatment algorithm for the prevention/management of headache in pediatric patients suffering from shunt over-drainage/slit ventricle syndrome.

General Recommendation:	
1. Almost always, even at initial shunt insertion, prefer the use of programmable valves with an integrated anti-siphon device. 2. In every case, we should carefully investigate the possibility of central catheter occlusion as the cause of recent-onset headache. In cases of established slit ventricle syndrome, the ventricular size is hardly expected to be enlarged, as in cases of sudden onset hydrocephalus that do not have as a substrate SVS.	
First step	Exclude other non-shunt related causes of headache (i.e., migraine).
Second step	In case of a headache compatible with shunt over-drainage, upgrade the opening valve pressure (differential pressure)
Third step	If the previous step proves to be inefficient and the patients valve lacks an ASD, insert an ASD in line with the valvular mechanism.
Fourth step	Upgrade the ASD pressure (in case it is adjustable) or replace the existing ASD with another with higher opening pressure.
Fifth step	Replace the valve with another one with a programmable ASD combined with a programmable valve and adjust/upgrade both of them.
Finally, always keep in mind that in cases where slit ventricle syndrome is established, ventricular dimensions are not expected to restore to normal. Our ultimate goal is to avoid/eliminate the incidence of headache and not the normalization of the radiological appearance of the ventricular system.	

4. Conclusions

The overall effect of headache disorders on individual patients, as well as on society itself, is extremely difficult to elucidate with clarity and constitutes a target for public health interventions that is difficult, albeit important, to be achieved [1]. Although there is a widespread disability intimately associated with pediatric headaches, this disorder remains under-diagnosed and, most importantly, under-treated and not appropriately managed.

Moreover, SVS is intimately related to persistent and difficult-to-manage headaches in the pediatric population [15,16]. The main issue that we have to overcome regarding SVS is that its treatment is currently based primarily on sparse anecdotal reports as, to the best of our knowledge, there are no large cases series published which report results and treatment outcomes based on a widely accepted treatment algorithm. Nowadays, our main goal is centered on attempts to control CSF over-drainage and improve cerebral compliance [11,47]. Nonetheless, SVS remains an intractable problem as its management has proved to be insufficient in a significant percentage of patients, which is a fact that cannot be ignored. A promising technical advancement that will help us to associate the clinical parameters of slit ventricle syndrome with the underlying pathology (reduced cerebral compliance)is the innovation of telemetric systems for ICP measurement [78]. We hope that these devices will offer us the possibility of dynamic ICP monitoring in the near future, thus improving our therapeutic armamentarium in terms of the prevention, diagnosis, and treatment of SVS.

Author Contributions: Conceptualization, D.P., M.G., E.B., S.K. and M.T.; methodology, D.P. and M.G.; software, E.B., S.K. and M.T.; validation, D.P., M.G., E.B., S.K. and M.T.; formal analysis, D.P.; investigation S.K. and M.T.; resources D.P. and M.G.; data curation D.P.; writing—original draft preparation D.P., M.G. and E.B., writing—review and editing D.P., M.G., E.B., S.K. and M.T.; visualization, D.P.; supervision, D.P.; project administration, D.P. and M.G.; funding acquisition, not applicable. All authors have read and agreed to the published version of the manuscript.

Funding: This research received no external funding.

Data Availability Statement: No new data were created or analyzed in this study. Data sharing is not applicable to this article.

Conflicts of Interest: The authors declare no conflicts of interest.

Abbreviations

CSF	Cerebrospinal fluid
OD	Over-drainage
VPS	Ventriculoperitoneal shunt
SVS	Slit ventricle syndrome
VAS	Ventriculoatrial shunt
ASD	Anti-siphon device
ETV	Endoscopic third ventriculostomy
EVD	External ventricular drainage
ICP	intracranial pressure

References

1. Onofri, A.; Pensato, U.; Rosignoli, C.; Wells-Gatnik, W.; Stanyer, E.; Ornello, R.; Chen, H.Z.; De Santis, F.; Torrente, A.; Mikulenka, P.; et al. Primary headache epidemiology in children and adolescents: A systematic review and meta-analysis. *J. Headache Pain* **2023**, *24*, 8. [CrossRef] [PubMed]
2. Alashqar, A.; Shuaibi, S.; Ahmed, S.F.; AlThufairi, H.; Owayed, S.; AlHamdan, F.; Alroughani, R.; Al-Hashel, J.Y. Impact of puberty in girls on prevalence of primary headache disorder among female schoolchildren in Kuwait. *Front. Neurol.* **2020**, *11*, 594 [CrossRef] [PubMed]
3. Özge, A.; Faedda, N.; Abu-Arafeh, I.; Gelfand, A.A.; Goadsby, P.J.; Cuvellier, J.C.; Valeriani, M.; Sergeev, A.; Barlow, K.; Uludüz, D.; et al. Experts' opinion about the primary headache diagnostic criteria of the ICHD-3rd edition beta in children and adolescents. *J. Headache Pain* **2017**, *18*, 109. [CrossRef] [PubMed]
4. Abu-Arafeh, I.; Razak, S.; Sivaraman, B.; Graham, C. Prevalence of headache and migraine in children and adolescents: A systematic review of population-based studies. *Dev. Med. Child Neurol.* **2010**, *52*, 1088–1097. [CrossRef]
5. Arruda, M.A.; Bigal, M.E. Behavioral and emotional symptoms and primary headaches in children: A population-based study *Cephalalgia* **2012**, *32*, 1093–1100. [CrossRef] [PubMed]
6. Onofri, A.; Olivieri, L.; Silva, P.; Bernassola, M.; Tozzi, E. Correlation between primary headaches and learning disabilities in children and adolescents. *Minerva Pediatr.* **2022**, *74*, 1–6. [CrossRef] [PubMed]
7. Pedersen, S.H.; Prein, T.H.; Ammar, A.; Grotenhuis, A.; Hamilton, M.G.; Hansen, T.S.; Kehler, U.; Rekate, H.; Thomale, U.-W.; Juhler, M. How to define CSF overdrainage: A systematic literature review. *Acta Neurochir.* **2023**, *165*, 429–441. [CrossRef] [PubMed]
8. Becker, D.P.; Nulsen, F.E. Control of hydrocephalus by valve-regulated venous shunt: Avoidance of complications in prolonged shunt maintenance. *J. Neurosurg.* **1968**, *28*, 215–226. [CrossRef] [PubMed]
9. Decq, P.; Barat, J.-L.; Duplessis, E.; Leguerinel, C.; Gendrault, P.; Keravel, Y. Shunt failure in adult hydrocephalus: Flow-controlled shunt versus differential pressure shunts—A cooperative study in 289 patients. *Surg. Neurol.* **1995**, *43*, 333–339. [CrossRef]
10. Pudenz, R.H.; Foltz, E.L. Hydrocephalus: Overdrainage by ventricular shunts. A review and recommendations. *Surg. Neurol.* **1991**, *35*, 200–212. [CrossRef]
11. Tschan, C.A.; Antes, S.; Huthmann, A.; Vulcu, S.; Oertel, J.; Wagner, W. Overcoming CSF overdrainage with the adjustable gravitational valve proSA. *Acta Neurochir.* **2014**, *156*, 767–776. [CrossRef] [PubMed]
12. Kajimoto, Y.; Ohita, T.; Miyake, H.; Matsukawa, M.; Ogawa, D.; Nagao, K.; Kuroiwa, T. Posture-related changes in the pressure environment of the ventriculoperitoneal shunt system. *J. Neurosurg.* **2000**, *93*, 614–617. [CrossRef]
13. Feletti, A.; D'avella, D.; Wikkelsø, C.; Klinge, P.; Hellström, P.; Tans, J.; Kiefer, M.; Meier, U.; Lemcke, J.; Paternò, V.; et al. Ventriculoperitoneal shunt complications in the European idiopathic normal pressure hydrocephalus multicenter study. *Oper Neurosurg.* **2019**, *17*, 97–102. [CrossRef] [PubMed]
14. Rekate, H.L. Classifcation of slit-ventricle syndromes using intracranial pressure monitoring. *Pediatr. Neurosurg.* **1993**, *19*, 15–20. [CrossRef]
15. Ros, B.; Iglesias, S.; Martín, Á.; Carrasco, A.; Ibáñez, G.; Arráez, M.A. Shunt overdrainage syndrome: Review of the literature *Neurosurg. Rev.* **2018**, *41*, 969–981. [CrossRef]
16. Ros, B.; Iglesias, S.; Linares, J.; Cerro, L.; Casado, J.; Arráez, M.A. Shunt overdrainage: Reappraisal of the syndrome and proposal for an integrative model. *J. Clin. Med.* **2021**, *10*, 3620. [CrossRef] [PubMed]
17. Desai, V.R.; Sadrameli, S.S.; Jenson, A.V.; Asante, S.K.; Daniels, B.; Trask, T.W.; Britz, G. Ventriculoperitoneal shunt complications in an adult population: A comparison of various shunt designs to prevent overdrainage. *Surg. Neurol. Int.* **2020**, *5*, 269. [CrossRef]
18. Khan, Q.U.; Wharen, R.E.; Grewal, S.S.; Thomas, C.S.; Deen, H.G.; Reimer, R.; Van Gerpen, J.A.; Crook, J.E.; Graf-Radford, N.R. Overdrainage shunt complications in idiopathic normal-pressure hydrocephalus and lumbar puncture opening pressure. *J. Neurosurg.* **2013**, *119*, 1498–1502. [CrossRef]
19. Trinh, V.T.; Duckworth, E.A.M. Revision to an adjustable non-siphon control valve in low pressure hydrocephalus: Therapeutic siphoning and a new perspective on NPH. *Clin. Neurol. Neurosurg.* **2013**, *115*, 175–178. [CrossRef]

20. Weinzweig, J.; Bartlett, S.P.; Chen, J.C.; Losee, J.; Sutton, L.; Duhaime, A.C.; Whitaker, L.A. Cranial vault expansion in the management of post-shunt craniosynostosis and slit ventricle syndrome. *Plast. Reconstr. Surg.* **2008**, *122*, 1171–1180. [CrossRef]
21. Chan, S.M.; Chodakiewitz, Y.G.; Maya, M.M.; Schievink, W.I.; Moser, F.G. Intracranial hypotension and cerebrospinal fluid leak. *Neuroimaging Clin. N. Am.* **2019**, *29*, 213–226. [CrossRef] [PubMed]
22. Kraemer, M.R.; Sandoval-Garcia, C.; Bragg, T.; Iskandar, B.J. Shunt-dependent hydrocephalus: Management style among members of the American Society of Pediatric Neurosurgeons. *J. Neurosurg. Pediatr.* **2017**, *20*, 216–224. [CrossRef] [PubMed]
23. Tan, K.; Meiri, A.; Mowrey, W.B.; Abbott, R.; Goodrich, J.T.; Sandler, A.L.; Suri, A.K.; Lipton, M.L.; Wagshul, M.E. Diffusion tensor imaging and ventricle volume quantifcation in patients with chronic shunt-treated hydrocephalus: A matched case-control study. *J. Neurosurg.* **2018**, *129*, 1611–1622. [CrossRef]
24. Chari, A.; Dasgupta, D.; Smedley, A.; Craven, C.; Dyson, E.; Matloob, S.; Thompson, S.; Thorne, L.; Toma, A.K.; Watkins, L. Intra-parenchymal intracranial pressure monitoring for hydrocephalus and cerebrospinal fuid disorders. *Acta Neurochir.* **2017**, *159*, 1967–1978. [CrossRef] [PubMed]
25. Norager, N.H.; Olsen, M.H.; Pedersen, S.H.; Riedel, C.S.; Czosnyka, M.; Juhler, M. Reference values for intracranial pressure and lumbar cerebrospinal fluid pressure: A systematic review. *Fluids Barriers CNS* **2021**, *18*, 19. [CrossRef]
26. Pedersen, S.H.; Lilja-Cyron, A.; Andresen, M.; Juhler, M. The relationship between intracranial pressure and age—Chasing age-related reference values. *World Neurosurg.* **2018**, *110*, e119–e123. [CrossRef]
27. Qvarlander, S.; Sundstrom, N.; Malm, J.; Eklund, A. Postural effects on intracranial pressure: Modeling and clinical evaluation. *J. Appl. Physiol.* **2013**, *115*, 1474–1480. [CrossRef]
28. Grunert, P.; Charalampaki, P.; Ayyad, A. Concept and treatment of hydrocephalus in the Greco-Roman and early Arabic Medicine. *Minim. Invasive Neurosurg.* **2007**, *50*, 253–264. [CrossRef]
29. Rachel, R.A. Surgical treatment of hydrocephalus: A historical perspective. *Pediatr. Neurosurg.* **1999**, *30*, 296–304. [CrossRef]
30. Kompaje, E.J.; Delwel, E.J. The first description of a device for repeated external ventricular drainage in the treatment of congenital hydrocephalus, invented in 1744 by Claude-Nicolas Le Cat. *Pediatr. Neurosurg.* **2003**, *39*, 10–13. [CrossRef]
31. Cheok, S.; Chen, J.; Lazareff, J. The truth and coherence behind the concept of overdrainage of cerebrospinal fluid in hydrocephalic patients. *Child's Nerv. Syst.* **2014**, *30*, 599–606. [CrossRef]
32. Strenger, L. Complications of ventriculovenous shunts. *J. Neurosurg.* **1963**, *20*, 219–224. [CrossRef] [PubMed]
33. Hayward, R. "Casey and Theo": The children who changed the face of "Water-on-the-brain". *Br. J. Neurosurg.* **2009**, *23*, 347–350. [CrossRef] [PubMed]
34. Fox, J.L.; McCullough, D.C.; Green, R.C. Effect of cerebrospinal fluid shunts on intracranial pressure and on cerebrospinal fluid dynamics 2. A new technique of pressure measurements: Results and concepts 3. A concept of hydrocephalus. *J. Neurol. Neurosurg. Psychiatry* **1973**, *36*, 302–312. [CrossRef]
35. Portnoy, H.D.; Schulte, R.R.; Fox, J.L.; Croissant, P.D.; Tripp, L. Antisiphon and reversible occlusion valves for shunting in hydrocephalus and preventing post-shunt subdural hematomas. *J. Neurosurg.* **1973**, *38*, 729–738. [CrossRef] [PubMed]
36. Chapman, P.H.; Cosman, E.R.; Arnold, M.A. The relationship between ventricular fluid pressure and body position in normal subjects and subjects with shunts: A telemetric study. *Neurosurgery* **1990**, *26*, 181–189. [CrossRef] [PubMed]
37. Niimura, M.; Takai, K.; Taniguchi, M. Postoperative epidural haematomas associated with hydrocephalus caused by intraoperative overdrainage of cerebrospinal fluid: Two case reports with a literature review of 19 cases. *BMJ Case Rep.* **2015**, *2015*, bcr2014206654. [CrossRef] [PubMed]
38. Niwa, R.; Oya, S.; Nakamura, T.; Hana, T.; Matsui, T. Rapid intracranial pressure drop as a cause for posterior reversible encephalopathy syndrome: Two case reports. *Surg. Neurol. Int.* **2017**, *8*, 103. [PubMed]
39. Weerakkody, R.A.; Czosnyka, M.; Schuhmann, M.U.; Schmidt, E.; Keong, N.; Santarius, T.; Pickard, J.D.; Czosnyka, Z. Clinical assessment of cerebrospinal fluid dynamics in hydrocephalus. Guide to interpretation based on observational study. *Acta Neurol. Scand.* **2011**, *124*, 85–98. [CrossRef]
40. Hart, M.G.; Czosnyka, M.; Czosnyka, Z.H.; Fernandes, H.M. Combined intracranial pressure monitoring and cerebrospinal fluid infusion study to guide management of slit ventricle syndrome. *Pediatr. Neurosurg.* **2013**, *49*, 113–118. [CrossRef]
41. Schuhmann, M.U.; Sood, S.; McAllister, J.P.; Jaeger, M.; Ham, S.D.; Czosnyka, Z.; Czosnyka, M. Value of overnight monitoring of intracranial pressure in hydrocephalic children. *Pediatr. Neurosurg.* **2008**, *44*, 269–279. [CrossRef] [PubMed]
42. Auricchio, A.M.; Bohnen, A.; Nichelatti, M.; Cenzato, M.; Talamonti, G. Management of slit ventricle syndrome: A single-center case series of 32 surgically treated patients. *World Neurosurg.* **2022**, *158*, e352–e361. [CrossRef] [PubMed]
43. Fernández-Méndez, R.; Richards, H.K.; Seeley, H.M.; Pickard, J.D.; Joannides, A.J. Current epidemiology of cerebrospinal fluid shunt surgery in the UK and Ireland (2004–2013). *J. Neurol. Neurosurg. Psychiatry* **2019**, *90*, 747–754. [CrossRef] [PubMed]
44. Aschoff, A.; Kremer, P.; Benesch, C.; Fruh, K.; Klank, A.; Kunze, S. Overdrainage and shunt technology. A critical comparison of programmable, hydrostatic and variable-resistance valves and flow-reducing devices. *Child's Nerv. Syst.* **1995**, *11*, 193–202. [CrossRef] [PubMed]
45. Hanlo, P.W.; Cinalli, G.; Vandertop, W.P.; Faber, J.A.J.; Bøgeskov, L.; Børgesen, S.E.; Boschert, J.; Chumas, P.; Eder, H.; Pople, I.K.; et al. Treatment of hydrocephalus determined by the European Orbis Sigma Valve II survey: A multicenter prospective 5-year shunt survival study in children and adults in whom a flow-regulating shunt was used. *J. Neurosurg.* **2003**, *99*, 52–57. [CrossRef] [PubMed]

46. Drake, J.M.; Kestle, J.R.; Milner, R.; Cinalli, G.; Boop, F.; Piatt, J., Jr.; Haines, S.; Schiff, S.J.; Cochrane, D.D.; Steinbok, P.; et al. Randomized trial of cerebrospinal fluid shunt valve design in pediatric hydrocephalus. *Neurosurgery* **1998**, *43*, 294–303; discussion: 303–305. [CrossRef]
47. Weinzierl, M.R.; Hans, F.-J.; Stoffel, M.; Oertel, M.F.; Korinth, M.C. Experience with a gravitational valve in the management of symptomatic overdrainage in children with shunts. *J. Neurosurg. Pediatr.* **2012**, *9*, 468–472. [CrossRef]
48. Gebert, A.-F.; Schulz, M.; Schwarz, K.; Thomale, U.-W. Long-term survival rates of gravity-assisted, adjustable differential pressure valves in infants with hydrocephalus. *J. Neurosurg. Pediatr.* **2016**, *17*, 544–551. [CrossRef]
49. Liniger, P.; Marchand, S.; Kaiser, G.L. Flow control versus antisiphon valves: Late results concerning slit ventricles and slit-ventricle syndrome. *Eur. J. Pediatr. Surg.* **2003**, *13* (Suppl. S1), S3–S6. [PubMed]
50. Antes, S.; Eymann, R.; Schmitt, M.; Kiefer, M. Pathophysiology of brainstem lesions due to over-drainage. *Acta Neurochir. Suppl.* **2012**, *113*, 177–180.
51. Fattal-Valevski, A.; Beni-Adani, L.; Constantini, S. Short-term dexamethasone treatment for symptomatic slit ventricle syndrome. *Child's Nerv. Syst.* **2005**, *21*, 981–984. [CrossRef] [PubMed]
52. Kan, P.; Walker, M.L.; Drake, J.M.; Kestle, J.R.W. Predicting slit-like ventricles in children on the basisof baseline characteristics at the time of shunt insertion. *J. Neurosurg.* **2007**, *106* (Suppl. S5), 347–349. [PubMed]
53. Beez, T.; Munoz-Bendix, C.; Ahmadi, S.A.; Messing-Jünger, M.; Steiger, H.-J.; Röhrig, A. Conservative and operative management of iatrogenic craniocerebral disproportion—A case-based review. *Child's Nerv. Syst.* **2019**, *35*, 19–27. [CrossRef] [PubMed]
54. Major, O.; Fedorcsák, I.; Sipos, L.; Hantos, P.; Kónya, E.; Dobronyi, I.; Paraicz, E. Slit-ventricle syndrome in shunt operated children. *Acta Neurochir.* **1994**, *127*, 69–72. [CrossRef] [PubMed]
55. Obana, W.G.; Raskin, N.H.; Cogen, P.H.; Szymanski, J.A.; Edwards, M.S. Antimigraine treatment for slit ventricle syndrome. *Neurosurgery* **1990**, *27*, 760–763; discussion: 763. [CrossRef] [PubMed]
56. Hoffman, H.J.; Tucker, W.S. Cephalocranial disproportion. A complication of the treatment of hydrocephalus in children. *Child's Brain* **1976**, *2*, 167–176. [PubMed]
57. Martínez-Lage, J.F.; Poza, M.; López, F. Arachnoid cyst as a complication of ventricular shunting. *Child's Nerv. Syst.* **1991**, *7*, 356–357. [CrossRef] [PubMed]
58. Schijman, E.; Peter, J.C.; Rekate, H.L.; Sgouros, S.; Wong, T.T. Management of hydrocephalus in posterior fossa tumors: How, what, when? *Child's Nerv. Syst.* **2004**, *20*, 192–194. [CrossRef] [PubMed]
59. Serlo, W.; Saukkonen, A.L.; Heikkinen, E.; von Wendt, L. The incidence and management of the slit ventricle syndrome. *Acta Neurochir.* **1989**, *99*, 113–116. [CrossRef]
60. Walker, M.L.; Fried, A.; Petronio, J. Diagnosis and treatment of the slit ventricle syndrome. *Neurosurg. Clin. N. Am.* **1993**, *4*, 707–714. [CrossRef]
61. Matsumoto, K.; Ohta, M.; Takeshita, I. Symptomatic spinal extramedullary mass lesion secondary to chronic overdrainage of ventricular fluid-case report. *Neurol. Med.-Chir.* **2002**, *42*, 140–142. [CrossRef]
62. Moayeri, N.N.; Henson, J.W.; Schaefer, P.W.; Zervas, N.T. Spinal dural enhancement on magnetic resonance imaging associated with spontaneous intracranial hypotension. Report of three cases and review of the literature. *J. Neurosurg.* **1998**, *88*, 912–918. [CrossRef]
63. Kobayashi, A.; Hashi, K. Secondary spinal canal stenosis associated with long-term ventriculoperitoneal shunting. *J. Neurosurg.* **1983**, *59*, 854–860. [CrossRef] [PubMed]
64. Nomura, S.; Fujii, M.; Kajiwara, K.; Ishihara, H.; Suehiro, E.; Goto, H.; Suzuki, M. Factors influencing spinal canal stenosis in patients with long-term controlled hydrocephalus treated with cerebrospinal fluid shunt. *Child's Nerv. Syst.* **2010**, *26*, 931–935. [CrossRef] [PubMed]
65. Yoon, S.J.; Oh, G.S.; Lee, S.J.; Lee, B.R.; Chun, J.-U.; Yu, I.K. Pneumocephalus in patients with orthostatic headache. *J. Clin. Neurol.* **2008**, *4*, 89–93. [CrossRef]
66. Chernov, M.F.; Kamikawa, S.; Yamane, F.; Ishihara, S.; Hori, T. Neurofiberscope-guided management of slit-ventricle syndrome due to shunt placement. *J. Neurosurg.* **2005**, *102* (Suppl. S3), 260–267. [CrossRef] [PubMed]
67. Steinbok, P.; Poskitt, K.J.; Cochrane, D.D.; Kestle, J.R. Prevention of postshunting ventricular asymmetry by transseptal placement of ventricular catheters. A randomized study. *Pediatr. Neurosurg.* **1994**, *21*, 59–64; discussion: 65. [CrossRef]
68. Rekate, H.L. Shunt-related headaches: The slit ventricle syndromes. *Child's Nerv. Syst.* **2008**, *24*, 423–430. [CrossRef]
69. Sandler, A.L.; Goodrich, J.T.; Daniels, L.B.; Biswas, A.; Abbott, R. Craniocerebral disproportion: A topicalreview and proposal toward a new definition, diagnosis, and treatment protocol. *Child's Nerv. Syst.* **2013**, *29*, 1997–2010. [CrossRef]
70. Canzi, G.; Auricchio, A.M.; Iacopino, G.; Cenzato, M.; Talamonti, G. Aesthetic cranial vault expansion in a child with slit ventricle syndrome and eumorphic face. *J. Craniofac. Surg.* **2019**, *30*, 2609–2613. [CrossRef]
71. Atalay, B.; Yilmaz, C.; Cekinmez, M.; Altinors, N.; Caner, H. Treatment of hydrocephalus with functionally isolated ventricles. *Acta Neurochir.* **2006**, *148*, 1293–1296. [CrossRef] [PubMed]
72. Laurence, K.M.; Coates, S. The natural history of hydrocephalus. Detailed analysis of 182 unoperated cases. *Arch. Dis. Child.* **1962**, *37*, 345–362. [CrossRef] [PubMed]
73. Butler, W.E.; Khan, S.A. The application of controlled intracranial hypertension in slit ventricle syndrome patients with obstructive hydrocephalus and shunt malfunction. *Pediatr. Neurosurg.* **2001**, *35*, 305–310. [CrossRef] [PubMed]

74. Khorasani, L.; Sikorski, C.W.; Frim, D.M. Lumbar CSF shunting preferentially drains the cerebral subarachnoid over the ventricular spaces: Implications for the treatment of slit ventricle syndrome. *Pediatr. Neurosurg.* **2004**, *40*, 270–276. [CrossRef] [PubMed]
75. Rekate, H.L. The slit ventricle syndrome: Advances based on technology and understanding. *Pediatr. Neurosurg.* **2004**, *40*, 259–263. [CrossRef] [PubMed]
76. Schatz, I.J. Orthostatic hypotension. I. Functional and neurogenic causes. *Arch. Intern. Med.* **1984**, *144*, 773–777. [CrossRef] [PubMed]
77. Winston, K.R.; French, B.; Bunn, J. Chronic debilitating headache in adults caused by craniocerebral disproportion: Treatment by cranial vault expansion. *Cureus* **2018**, *10*, e2187. [CrossRef] [PubMed]
78. Pedersen, S.H.; Henriksen, K.A.; Gustafsen, S.D.; Hansen, T.S.; Guldager, R.; Juhler, M. Telemetric ICP monitoring in children: A national questionnaire-based study. *Child's Nerv. Syst.* **2024**, *8*, 1–9. [CrossRef]

MDPI AG
Grosspeteranlage 5
4052 Basel
Switzerland
Tel.: +41 61 683 77 34

Children Editorial Office
E-mail: children@mdpi.com
www.mdpi.com/journal/children